W9-AHE-318

Maternal-Newborn Nursing

Consulting Editor
Alice B. Pappas, Ph.D., R.N.
Assistant Professor
Baylor University School of Nursing
Dallas, Texas

Reviewers
Andrea O. Hollingsworth, Ph.D., R.N.
Associate Professor and Director of Undergraduate Program
College of Nursing
Villanova University
Villanova, Pennsylvania

Janice C. Livingston, R.N., M.Ed., M.S., A.R.N.P.
Professor
Central Florida Community College
Ocala, Florida

Developed for Delmar Publishers Inc. by Visual Education Corporation,
Princeton, New Jersey.
Publisher: David Gordon
Sponsoring Editor: Patricia Casey
Project Director: Susan J. Garver
Production Supervisor: Amy Davis
Proofreading Management: Christine Osborne
Word Processing: Cynthia C. Feldner
Composition: Maxson Crandall, Lisa Evans-Skopas
Cover Designer: Paul C. Uhl, DESIGNASSOCIATES
Text Designer: Circa 86

For information, address
Delmar Publishers Inc.
3 Columbia Circle
Box 15015
Albany, New York 12212.

Printed in the United States of America
Published simultaneously in Canada by Nelson Canada, a division of
The Thomson Corporation

10 9 8 7 6 5 4 3 2 1

Library of Congress Cataloging-in-Publication Data

Maternal-newborn nursing / consulting editor, Alice B. Pappas;
reviewers, Andrea O. Hollingsworth, Janice C. Livingston.
p.   cm. — (NSNA review series)
Developed for Delmar Publishers Inc. by Visual Education Corporation.
ISBN 0-8273-5674-9
1. Maternity nursing.   I. Pappas, Alice B.   II. Hollingsworth, Andrea O.
III. Livingston, Janice C.   IV. Visual Education Corporation.   V. Series.
[DNLM: 1. Maternal-Child Nursing—outlines.   WY 18 M4255 1994]
RG951.M3148   1994
610.73´678—dc20
DNLM/DLC
for Library of Congress   93-37630
                                                                 CIP

Titles in Series

Maternal-Newborn Nursing

Pediatric Nursing

Nursing Pharmacology

Medical-Surgical Nursing

Psychiatric Nursing

Gerontologic Nursing
(available in 1995)

Health Assessment/Physical Assessment
(available in 1995)

Series Advisory Board

Series Review Board

Contents

Notice to the Reader

The publisher, editors, advisors, and reviewers do not warrant or guarantee any of the products described herein nor have they performed any independent analysis in connection with any of the product information contained herein. The publisher, editors, advisors, and reviewers do not assume, and each expressly disclaims, any obligation to obtain and include information other than that provided to them by the manufacturer.

The reader is expressly warned to consider and adopt all safety precautions that might be indicated by the activities described herein and to avoid all potential hazards. By following the instructions contained herein, the reader willingly assumes all risks in connection with such instructions.

The publisher, editors, advisors, and reviewers make no representations or warranties of any kind, including but not limited to the warranties of fitness for particular purpose or merchantability, nor are any such representations implied with respect to the material set forth herein, and the publisher, editors, advisors, and reviewers take no responsibility with respect to such material. The publisher, editors, advisors, and reviewers shall not be liable for any special, consequential, or exemplary damages resulting, in whole or in part, from readers' use of, or reliance upon, this material.

A conscientious effort has been made to ensure that the drug information and recommended dosages in this book are accurate and in accord with accepted standards at the time of publication. However, pharmacology is a rapidly changing science, so readers are advised, before administering any drug, to check the package insert provided by the manufacturer for the recommended dose, for contraindications for administration, and for added warnings and precautions. This recommendation is especially important for new, infrequently used, or highly toxic drugs.

CPR standards are subject to frequent change due to ongoing research. The American Heart Association can verify changing CPR standards when applicable. Recommended Schedules for Immunization are also subject to frequent change. The American Academy of Pediatrics, Committee on Infectious Diseases can verify changing recommendations.

Preface

The NSNA Review Series is a multiple-volume series designed to help nursing students review course content and prepare for course tests.

Chapter elements include:

Overview—lists the main topic headings for the chapter

Nursing Highlights—gives significant nursing care concepts relevant to the chapter

Glossary—features key terms used in the chapter that are not defined within the chapter

Enhanced Outline—consists of short, concise phrases, clauses, and sentences that summarize the main topics of course content; focuses on nursing care and the nursing process; includes the following elements:
- *Client Teaching Checklists:* shaded boxes that feature important issues to discuss with clients; designed to help students prepare client education sections of nursing care plans
- *Nurse Alerts:* shaded boxes that provide information that is of critical importance to the nurse, such as danger signs or emergency measures connected with a particular condition or situation
- *Locators:* finding aids placed across the top of the page that indicate the main outline section that is being covered on a particular 2-page spread within the context of other main section heads
- *Textbook reference aids:* boxes labeled "See text pages ____," which appear in the margin next to each main head, to be used by students to list the page numbers in their textbook that cover the material presented in that section of the outline
- *Cross references:* references to other parts of the outline, which identify the relevant section of the outline by using the numbered and lettered outline levels (e.g., "same as section I,A,1,b" or "see section II,B,3")

Chapter Tests—review and reinforce chapter material through questions in a format similar to that of the National Council Licensure Examination for Registered Nurses (NCLEX-RN); answers follow the questions and contain rationales for both correct and incorrect answers

Comprehensive Test—appears at the end of the book and includes items that review material from each chapter

1

Introduction

NURSING HIGHLIGHTS

1. Family theory provides a framework for the nurse to understand how families function and to provide adequate nursing care.
2. Nurse must practice within a defined scope of practice and adhere to predetermined standards of care.
3. Nurse is responsible for knowing standards of care and maintaining clinical competence to meet those standards.
4. Nurse is responsible for supporting clients' rights to privacy, informed consent, and confidentiality.
5. Nurse who has an ethical dilemma has the right to refuse to participate in or perform certain procedures, unless client's life is in danger.
6. Nurse should analyze in advance her/his own moral, religious, and ethical position about clinical dilemmas that might arise in practice.

ENHANCED OUTLINE

See text pages
_____

I. Maternal-newborn nursing

A. Definition: delivery of professional health care to client and client's family throughout the experience of childbearing

B. Practice settings: hospital maternity units, birth centers, doctors' offices, public health department clinics, family planning centers

C. Types of maternal-newborn nurses
   1. Registered nurse
      a) Graduate of an accredited basic nursing program
      b) Passed the National Council Licensure Examination for Registered Nurses (NCLEX-RN)
      c) Currently licensed by the state
      d) Provides basic nursing care
   2. Maternity nurse practitioner
      a) Received specialized education through master's degree or certification program
      b) Has expanded role, providing prenatal care to client and family in uncomplicated pregnancies (conducts physical examinations, orders and interprets tests, makes clinical diagnoses, and initiates treatment in consultation with physician)
   3. Family nurse practitioner
      a) Has same training and responsibilities as maternity nurse practitioner
      b) Can also provide postdelivery care for baby
   4. Maternity clinical nurse specialist
      a) Received master's degree
      b) Can handle problems associated with pregnancy; may have subspecialty, such as maternal diabetes or Rh sensitivity in pregnant woman
      c) May serve as consultant to registered nurses working in maternal-newborn field
    5. Certified nurse-midwife (CNM)
      a) Registered nurse with special education in midwifery through master's degree or certification program
      b) Certified according to requirements of the American College of Nurse-Midwives
      c) Independently manages care of healthy woman and newborn during normal pregnancy and delivery and throughout postpartum period
      d) Provides well-woman care

II. Family issues: Maternal-newborn nursing care is based on a family-centered approach.

See text pages

A. Family structures
1. Nuclear family: husband, wife, and children who live in a common household
2. Nuclear dyad: husband and wife who live alone; also called beginning family
3. Single-parent family: 1 head of household and children; increasingly common structure
4. Extended (3-generation) family: 1 or more grandparents living with a single-parent family or a nuclear family
5. Blended (reconstituted) family: parents/stepparents living with children from prior marriage and from current marriage
6. Kin network: 2 or more nuclear families or unmarried households living in close proximity
7. Single adult: unmarried adult living alone; sometimes not considered a family configuration

B. Family functions: Families need to perform certain tasks to assure survival of family as a unit and individuals within the unit.
1. Affective function: The family must meet the emotional needs of each member to promote the development of healthy personalities through mutual bonds of affection and trust.
2. Reproductive function: The family must provide for perpetuation and continuity within the family system and society.
3. Financial function: The family must earn money; determine allocation of resources for food, shelter, and clothing; and assure financial security.
4. Sociocultural function: The family must socialize children, teaching them rules of behavior, moral values, and social, cultural, and religious traditions.
5. Coping function: The family must teach skills, attitudes, and knowledge to allow members to adapt to stress and crises.

C. Changes in family system during childbearing
1. Structure: change in configuration of family
2. Power: changes in designation of authority within the family and in allocation of decision-making tasks
3. Boundaries: use of community sources and other resources outside family
4. Feelings: growth of maternal and paternal feelings and change in sexual and romantic feelings between couple
5. Roles: changes in division of labor in child-rearing tasks, wage earning, and household tasks
6. Communication: change in patterns between couple and between couple and close friends and relatives
7. Intergenerational patterns: adjustments to roles of grandparents and siblings

D. Influences on family's attitudes toward pregnancy and childbearing
   1. Culture: Pregnancy and childbearing have different meanings and behavioral expectations according to the cultural and ethnic background of the family.
   2. Socioeconomic status: Social and economic status affects family lifestyles, health practices, use of health services, and motivation for having children.
   3. Environment: Families are influenced by their living conditions, by relatives and friends, and by their community settings and religious and governmental institutions.

E. Nursing implications for treating the family unit during the childbearing cycle: In a family unit, the function of each member affects both the individual and the family; likewise, all members are affected by dysfunction within the family.
   1. Nursing assessment techniques
      a) Assess the family configuration, and obtain names, ages, and genders of all family members.
      b) Obtain health histories.
      c) Assess health beliefs and health practices that are based on culture, religion, and social status.
      d) Assess family functioning and home environment by asking questions and observing communication patterns and roles of family members.
   2. Nursing diagnosis and planning procedures
      a) Diagnoses should be developed from assessment data, keeping in mind the goals and needs of the family.
      b) Goals must be arranged according to priority.
      c) Health care workers and agencies that can help the family should be determined.
   3. Nursing intervention concerns
      a) Care must be specific to individual needs of family.
      b) Short- and long-term goals must be considered.
   4. Nursing evaluation techniques
      a) Family should be involved in evaluation.
      b) Reevaluations should be done as needed.

See text pages
_____

III. Legal and ethical considerations in maternal-newborn nursing

A. Scope of nursing care: Professional conduct requires that the nurse observe state nurse practice acts and standards of care.
   1. Nurse practice acts are state laws that determine education standards, licensing requirements, and minimum standards of care.

2. Laws and regulations indicate limits of nursing practice and identify appropriate functions and actions for nurses.
3. Professional nurses must observe at least the minimum standard of care.
   a) Standard of care is the code of expected behavior or performance for a professional nurse.
   b) Standard of care is described as the average degree of skill, care, and diligence that would be performed under similar circumstances by nurses with a similar background, training, and experience.
   c) Standards of care are established by these means:
      (1) Professional organizations such as American Nurses' Association or Association of Women's Health, Obstetric, and Neonatal Nurses (AWHONN) (formerly NAACOG)
      (2) State laws and regulations that define the scope of practice
      (3) Hospitals and institutions that employ nurses
   d) Nurses must provide care and document that care according to AWHONN standards and hospital protocol.

B. Bases for malpractice (negligence by a professional)
   1. Negligence occurs when nurse had duty to client, failed to fulfill duty, and caused harm to occur as a result of the breach.
   2. Breach of duty occurs when nurse performs unauthorized act, fails to act, or carries out authorized act improperly.
   3. Malpractice may lead to loss of license and to lawsuit.
   4. Nurse has liability in negligence suits.
      a) Nurses are responsible for the direct and indirect results caused by their actions.
      b) Nurse does not have to intend harm.
      c) Increasing independent practice of nursing has expanded nursing liability.
         (1) Physician or hospital is no longer always the liable party for nursing actions.
         (2) Every nurse should consider carrying personal liability insurance.
      d) Nurse has legal obligation to know and understand standards of care.
      e) Nurse is legally accountable for care she/he gives and for reporting inferior or inappropriate care given by members of the health team.
      f) Nurse is responsible for maintaining professional competency and for being current on practices and standards of care. Ignorance is not an excuse.

C. Clients' rights
   1. Right to privacy: Only those responsible for a client's care should examine her or discuss her case.

2. Informed consent: Client must give consent for all treatment, after being informed about a procedure, its benefits, risks, and alternatives.
   a) Responsibility for obtaining consent should rest with the individual performing the procedure.
   b) Information should be thorough, geared to educational level of the client, and well documented, including client's refusal of treatment.
3. Confidentiality: Communications that occur between the client and the nurse are confidential but are not protected by the law of privilege in most states; information from the communication can be subpoenaed.

D. Ethical and legal issues
   1. Abortion
      a) Ethical issue: conflict between a client's right to make choices about her body versus the fetus's right to life
      b) Legal issue: Although *Roe v. Wade* legalized abortion in 1973, it is currently being challenged to be overruled or to have restrictions.
      c) Nurse's responsibility
         (1) Nurse has the right to refuse to assist with the procedure if abortion is contrary to individual moral or ethical beliefs, unless client's life is in danger. Best course of action is not to accept employment in a facility that provides abortions.
         (2) Some institutions have a "conscience clause" outlining the policy for refusal to perform or assist with the abortion procedure.
   2. Neonatal intensive care
      a) Ethical and legal issues
         (1) What factors should be considered to determine viability?
         (2) Is treatment justifiable even though it may be futile and painful?
         (3) Who should decide whether high-risk preterm newborns are treated and the extent of the treatment?
         (4) Should invasive procedures that may produce disease or defects be employed?
      b) Nurse's responsibility
         (1) Nurse should be familiar with institutional policy concerning "no code" or withholding of treatment.
         (2) Nurse should encourage family's active participation in decision making.
         (3) Nurse should know how to access support for ethical concerns (i.e., from hospital ethics committee).
         (4) Nurse should discuss beliefs about treatment with other members of health care team.

3. Maternal care
   a) Ethical issue: conflict between the welfare of the fetus and a client's right to refuse to comply with medical recommendations that would benefit fetus
   b) Legal issue: Conflict centers on how far laws should extend to compel pregnant women to receive medical or surgical treatment for the benefit of the fetus; court cases and American College of Obstetricians and Gynecologists have acknowledged that every reasonable effort should be made to protect fetus while considering pregnant woman's autonomy.
   c) Nurse's responsibility: Nurse should rely on educating, counseling, and encouraging client to modify high-risk behavior.
4. Alternate conception methods (e.g., in vitro fertilization, artificial insemination with a donor, surrogacy)
   a) Ethical issues
      (1) For in vitro fertilization: how embryos that are not implanted should be handled
      (2) For in vitro fertilization, artificial insemination with donor, and surrogacy: parental rights and responsibilities of biological versus sociological parent; view that these procedures tamper with reproductive process; controversy of payment to sperm donor or surrogate mother
   b) Nurse's responsibility
      (1) Nurse should clarify personal beliefs about conception technology.
      (2) Nurse should provide factual information and emotional support to clients undergoing an alternate conception procedure.

1. Nancy N., R.N., is a certified nurse-midwife (CNM). Which of the following clients would you expect her to provide care for?

   a. Mary, age 30, nulligravida with acute asthma

   b. Juanita, age 28, in her second pregnancy, with no complications

   c. Helene, age 27, in her third pregnancy, with hydramnios

   d. Molly, age 14, nullipara with mild pregnancy-induced hypertension (PIH)

2. Ms. Marconi, R.N., M.S., is qualified to serve as a consultant to other nurses in the area of pregnant diabetes. She is called a:

   a. Maternity nurse practitioner.

   b. Family nurse practitioner.

   c. Clinical nurse specialist.

   d. Physician's assistant.

3. Bob and Sharon are married and have 4 children. Of these children, 2 are from Bob's previous marriage. This is an example of a(n):

   a. Extended family.

   b. Nuclear family.

   c. Blended family.

   d. Nuclear dyad.

4. Bob and Sharon bring their children to church each Sunday and have the children participate in Sunday school activities. This is an example of which type of family function?

   a. Coping

   b. Affective

   c. Financial

   d. Sociocultural

5. Which of the following is characteristic of the Native American culture?

   a. Most Native Americans deliver their babies at home.

   b. The elder members of the tribe are isolated.

   c. The family unit is an extended family.

   d. Female babies are not valued as highly as male babies.

6. Nurse Gotshalk is caring for Rita postpartum day 1. Rita asks the nurse for pain medication for relief of episiotomy pain. Without a physician's order, the nurse gives Rita 2 plain Tylenol to relieve pain. This is an example of:

   a. Breach of duty.

   b. Breach of right to privacy.

   c. Wrongful intent.

   d. Risk management.

7. Nurse practice acts are state statutes that have which of the following characteristics?

   a. They define the scope of nursing activities.

   b. They are uniform for all states.

   c. They define patients' rights.

   d. They provide specific ethical guidelines for nurses.

8. Carolyn is a nurse on the postpartum unit. As she enters Mei-ling Wu's room, Mrs. Wu, who is visibly upset and angry, states, "My doctor has explained my surgery and is trying to pressure me into signing the consent form, but I need more time to think it over." Which of the following general areas of patients' rights is possibly being violated?

   a. The right of self-determination

   b. The right to adequate medical care

   c. The right to information

   d. The right to privacy

9. Two nurses from the Women's Health Clinic are eating lunch when one says, "Guess who came in today for an abortion." The coworker's response should be:

a. "Tell me, who?"
b. "Perhaps this isn't the place to talk about it."
c. "I really don't need to know."
d. "Anyone I know?"

10. Mrs. Harbison, age 29, is scheduled for a cesarean birth. Dr. Kaufman, her obstetrician, tells the nurse to obtain the consent for surgery from Mrs. Harbison. The nurse's best response to Dr. Kaufman is:

a. "I'll get it right away, Dr. Kaufman."
b. "I'll have to wait for her husband to be present."
c. "Dr. Kaufman, only you have authority to obtain consent."
d. "Dr. Kaufman, why can't you do it?"

11. Keshia Johnson, R.N., is assigned to a client who is scheduled for an elective second-trimester abortion. Abortion is contrary to Nurse Johnson's moral and ethical beliefs. The best action for Nurse Johnson to take is to:

a. Care for the client.
b. Ask for a different assignment.
c. Demand to be transferred to another unit for the day.
d. Call her pastor for advice.

12. Mrs. Anderson, nulligravida, has an infertility history related to endometriosis, which has destroyed her tubal function and restricts uterine implantation. Mr. Anderson's sperm are viable and motile. The couple have decided to contract with a woman named Marilyn who will bear their child for the sum of $15,000. This arrangement is called:

a. Surrogate childbearing.
b. Collaborative parenting.
c. Adoption.
d. Gamete intrafallopian transfer (GIFT).

1. **Correct answer is b.** Certified nurse-midwives provide independent care for women with normal pregnancies and for normal newborns.

   a. CNMs do not provide medical care for acute asthma. Such a client would be seen by a medical doctor.
   c and **d.** CNMs do not provide care for pregnant women who have these types of complications.

2. **Correct answer is c.** The clinical nurse specialist holds a master's degree and can handle problems associated with pregnancy or subspecialties such as maternal diabetes. This person often serves as a consultant to other nurses as they plan care for women with problem pregnancies.

   a and **b.** A maternity nurse practitioner or family nurse practitioner may have a master's degree or have received additional education through continuing education programs. Practitioners have an expanded role and provide client and family care in uncomplicated pregnancies and initiate treatment in consultation with a physician.
   d. A physician's assistant (PA) has received technical training from a physician and works under legal license of a physician; PAs are not trained or qualified to work as consultants to nurses.

3. **Correct answer is c.** A blended family consists of parents and stepparents living with children from prior marriages and from current marriage.

   a. Extended family consists of one or more grandparents living with a single-parent family or a nuclear family.
   b. Nuclear family consists of husband, wife, and children who live in a common household.
   d. Nuclear dyad consists of a husband and wife who live alone.

4. **Correct answer is d.** Families need to perform certain tasks to assure survival of the family unit. When parents socialize children and teach them moral values and religious traditions, they are carrying out sociocultural functions.

   a. Those tasks related to teaching children to adapt to stress and crises are called coping functions.
   b. When a family meets emotional needs and gives affection and trust, it is fulfilling an affective function.
   c. The function of a family to earn money and to provide food, clothing, and so on, is called the financial function.

5. **Correct answer is c.** The Native American family is an extended one, often comprised of grandparents, aunts, and uncles.

   a. Most Native Americans deliver their babies in hospitals.
   b. Elder members are held in high regard.
   d. All children are considered assets.

6. **Correct answer is a.** A breach of duty occurs when a nurse performs unauthorized acts, fails to act, or carries out an authorized act improperly.

   b. Nurse Gotshalk's action does not involve a privacy issue.
   c. Nurse Gotshalk did not exhibit wrongful intent or decide to harm the client; she gave the Tylenol to relieve pain.
   d. Risk management is an administrative function of a health care facility to identify and eliminate risk of injury to those at the facility.

7. **Correct answer is a.** Nurse practice acts are laws that define nursing practice (i.e., education standards, licensing requirements, and minimal standards of care).

   b. Nurse practice acts vary from state to state.

   c. Patients' rights are not provided for in nurse practice acts; they can be found in *A Patient's Bill of Rights*.
   d. Specific ethical guidelines for nurses can be found in documents such as *Code for Nurses* and in findings of hospital ethics boards.

8. **Correct answer is a.** Clients have the right to determine their future health care. They should not be pressured or coerced in any way.

   b. Mrs. Wu's right to adequate medical care is not being violated in this situation.
   c. Mrs. Wu seems to have the right information but needs time to make her decision.
   d. Mrs. Wu's situation does not relate to any privacy issues.

9. **Correct answer is c.** Only those individuals directly caring for a client should discuss the client. Clients have a right to privacy. Nurses have a responsibility to ensure confidentiality. In this case, the coworker really does not need to know who came into the clinic for an abortion.

   a and d. Answers to either of these questions would be a direct break in client confidentiality.
   b. There is no correct place to discuss clients for whom the nurse is not responsible.

10. **Correct answer is c.** Responsibility for obtaining consent should rest with the individual performing the surgery.

    a. It is not the nurse's responsibility to obtain the consent.
    b. Mrs. Harbison is of legal age and can sign her own consent form. Her husband need not be present.
    d. This is an unprofessional response that could put Dr. Kaufman in a defensive position. This reply would not facilitate a team approach.

11. **Correct answer is b.** A nurse has the right to refuse to care for a client when abortion is contrary to the nurse's moral or ethical beliefs, unless the client's life is in danger. Asking for a different assignment would be appropriate.

a. The nurse does not need to care for the client in this situation. It may be best for both the client and the nurse that someone with similar ethical or moral beliefs provides the care.
c. Demanding to be transferred to another unit is unprofessional. Perhaps the nurse's best course of action would be to seek employment in a facility or on a station where abortion care is not provided.
d. A call to her pastor would not be appropriate while on duty. Perhaps Nurse Johnson would benefit from a discussion with her pastor later.

12. **Correct answer is a.** In surrogate child-bearing, a woman agrees to bear a child for a couple who are unable to have a child of their own.

b. Collaborative parenting does not fit this situation. Once Marilyn has the baby, she relinquishes the child to the Andersons.
c. This is not a traditional adoptive situation, although the wife of the biologic father adopts the child carried by the surrogate.
d. Gamete intrafallopian transfer is used in women with at least 1 functioning fallopian tube. Multiple follicles are obtained via laparoscopy and transferred with sperm into the fallopian tubes.

2

Reproductive System and Sexuality

NURSING HIGHLIGHTS

1. Symptoms of menstrual disorders may be improved by self-care related to diet, exercise, rest, and stress reduction.
2. Reproductive activity is an interaction of reproductive structures, the central nervous system, and endocrine glands.
3. Sexuality must be considered in the context of an individual's life, including cultural background, education, religion, and personal choices.
4. Nurse must be aware of his/her own feelings, values, and beliefs about sexuality in order to effectively provide sexual health care to clients.
5. Nurse should anticipate that clients' feelings and values about sex may not be the same as his/her own.

corpus luteum—"yellow body" that ruptured ovarian follicle develops into after ovum is discharged at ovulation; secretes progesterone

dyspareunia—painful intercourse

endometrium—lining of uterus

gamete—mature male or female germ cell (sperm or ovum)

gonadotropin—hormone that stimulates the function of the testes and ovaries

graafian follicle—fully developed ovarian sac containing ripe ovum

menarche—onset of menstrual function

ENHANCED OUTLINE

I. Male reproductive system

See text pages
_____

A. External genitalia
  1. Penis: elongated organ of copulation and urination
     a) Shaft contains erectile tissue: paired corpora cavernosa and corpus spongiosum (which encloses urethra).
     b) End is sensitive structure called glans penis.
  2. Scrotum: pouch behind penis
     a) Has 2 compartments, each with testis, epididymis, and vas deferens
     b) Maintains temperature to protect testes and sperm

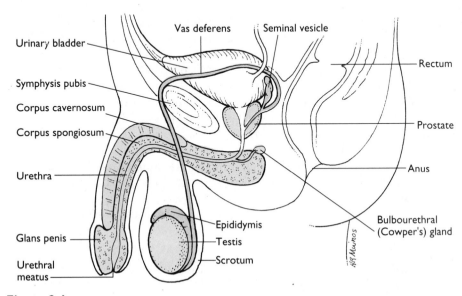

Figure 2-1
Male Reproductive System

   B. Internal genitalia
     1. Testes: organs of spermatogenesis and hormone production
      a) Seminiferous tubules produce sperm cells.
      b) Leydig's (interstitial) cells produce and release male sex hormone testosterone.
      c) Sertoli cells nourish and protect developing sperm.
     2. Ducts
      a) Epididymis: reservoir for sperm
      b) Vas deferens: duct that propels sperm from epididymis through ejaculatory duct to urethra
      c) Urethra: passageway for semen and urine from body
     3. Accessory structures
      a) Seminal vesicles, prostate, and bulbourethral (Cowper's) glands
      b) Secrete fluid and nutrients for sperm

   C. Function of male hormone testosterone
     1. Main role: production of sperm (spermatogenesis)
     2. Also establishes and maintains male secondary sex characteristics

   D. Source of testosterone: production stimulated by luteinizing hormone (LH) from anterior pituitary gland

II. Female reproductive system

See text pages
_____

   A. External genitalia (called vulva or pudendum)
     1. Mons pubis (mons veneris): subcutaneous fatty tissue covered with pubic hair; protects pelvic bones
     2. Labia majora: folds of adipose tissue forming internal borders of vulva; sensitive to stimuli
     3. Labia minora: soft tissue within labia majora; lubricate vulva, secrete bacteria-fighting substance, are sensitive to stimuli
     4. Clitoris: organ located posteriorly to mons pubis; highly sensitive to sexual stimulation
     5. Vestibule: contains urethral opening (urethral meatus), vaginal opening (introitus), hymen, ducts of Bartholin's glands, and ducts of Skene's glands
     6. Perineum: area between vagina and anus; contains muscles that support pelvis

   B. Internal genitalia
     1. Vagina (also known as birth canal): provides passage for sperm, fetus, and menstrual products
     2. Uterus: muscular, pear-shaped, thick-walled organ composed of corpus, isthmus, and cervix; nourishes and contains embryo and fetus during development

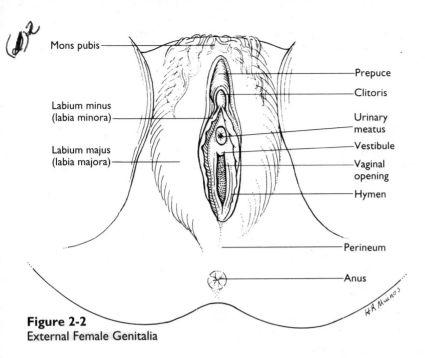

Figure 2-2
External Female Genitalia

Labels in figure:
Mons pubis
Labium minus (labia minora)
Labium majus (labia majora)
Prepuce
Clitoris
Urinary meatus
Vestibule
Vaginal opening
Hymen
Perineum
Anus

3. Cervix: canal-shaped structure that connects uterus and vagina; stretches during labor and delivery
4. Fallopian tubes: carry ovum from ovary to uterus; site of fertilization
5. Ovaries: provide ovum for fertilization monthly; source of hormones
6. Bony pelvis: made up of 2 hip bones, sacrum, and coccyx
   a) Hip bones (also called innominate bones) contain ilium, ischium, and pubis.
   b) Pelvic sections are divided at inlet, or brim.
      (1) False pelvis: supports pregnant uterus and directs fetus into true pelvis
      (2) True pelvis: forms bony limits of the birth canal
         (a) Parts: inlet, midpelvis, outlet
         (b) Importance of diameters of inlet, midpelvis, and outlet and of curvature (or axis) of cavity: These measurements determine ability of fetus to pass from uterus through birth canal.

C. Functions of female hormones
   1. Estrogen: responsible for maturation of ovarian follicles and for proliferation of endometrium; also establishes and maintains female secondary sex characteristics
   2. Progesterone: prepares endometrium to receive and nourish fertilized ovum; also relaxes uterine muscles
   3. Follicle stimulating hormone (FSH): stimulates development of graafian follicle
   4. Luteinizing hormone (LH): brings about final ripening of graafian follicle and ovulation

D. Sources of female hormone secretion
1. Pituitary gland, under regulation of hypothalamus, releases LH and FSH to stimulate ovaries.
2. Ovaries secrete estrogen and progesterone under the influence of LH and FSH.

E. Female reproductive cycle
1. Ovarian cycle
   a) Follicular phase: Ovarian follicles mature under influence of FSH and estrogen; LH surge causes ovulation. (days 1–14)
   b) Luteal phase: Ovum is discharged from mature follicle; corpus luteum develops under influence of LH, producing high levels of progesterone and some estrogen. (days 15–28)
2. Menstrual cycle (occurs simultaneously with ovarian cycle)
   a) Menstrual phase: Endometrium is shed during menstruation; estrogen levels are low. (days 1–5)
   b) Proliferative phase: Endometrium grows; ovarian follicle matures and ovulation occurs; estrogen levels rise sharply just before ovulation. (days 6–14)
   c) Secretory phase: Estrogen declines rapidly, and progesterone increases to enhance endometrial growth. (days 15–26)
   d) Ischemic phase: Corpus luteum degenerates, causing estrogen and progesterone levels to drop. (days 27–28)

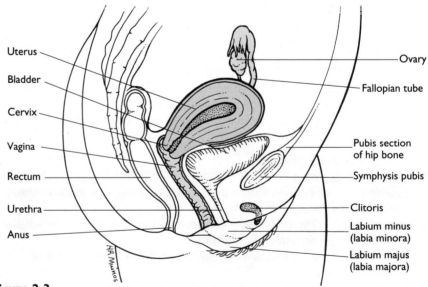

Figure 2-3
Internal Female Genitalia

F. Menstrual disorders
1. Dysmenorrhea: painful menstruation
a) Primary: no organic disease
b) Secondary: presence of disease in pelvis (e.g., endometriosis)
2. Premenstrual syndrome (PMS): recurrent, cyclic symptoms (e.g., irritability, fluid retention, headache, nervousness) that occur 7–10 days before menses and improve after menstrual flow begins
3. Cycle variations
a) Amenorrhea: absence of menses
(1) Primary: never menstruated; caused by structural, congenital, or endocrine abnormalities
(2) Secondary: cessation of menses; caused by pregnancy, oral contraceptives, tumors, cysts, hormonal imbalance, or stress
b) Anovulation: absence of ovulation with symptoms of irregular cycles, no menstrual distress and, often, heavy bleeding
(1) Primary: caused by pituitary or hypothalamic disorder, adrenal gland disorder, nutritional deficiency, or stress
(2) Secondary: caused by pituitary or hypothalamic disorder, ovarian disease, chronic illness, or drug use
4. Dysfunctional uterine bleeding: presence of heavy, light, or irregular bleeding; usually caused by endocrine dysfunction that causes failure of normal cyclic changes in endometrium

III. Physiology of sexual response

See text pages
_____

A. General processes in males and females
1. Vasocongestion: dilatation of blood vessels and congestion
2. Myotonia: increased muscle tension, followed by rhythmic muscle contractions

B. Phases of response cycle
1. Excitement (foreplay): in female, vaginal lubrication; in male, penile erection
2. Plateau (entry and coitus): engorgement of vagina and labia and clitoral retraction; elevation of testes and distension of urethra with semen
3. Orgasm (climax): in female, rhythmic muscle contractions of clitoris, vagina, and uterus; in male, contraction of penis and ejaculation of semen
4. Resolution (relaxation): return to unaroused state

C. Differences in response patterns of males and females
1. Some responses are the same for men and women: sex flush, muscle tension, and increases in heart rate and blood pressure.
2. Man and woman may reach each phase of response cycle at different times, affecting occurrence of simultaneous orgasm.
3. Response of females may vary from one sexual experience to another; male response is relatively constant each time.
4. Women are capable of multiple orgasms; men experience refractory phase during which they cannot have an erection.

I. Male reproductive system	II. Female reproductive system	III. Physiology of sexual response	IV. Psychologic influences on sexual response	V. Essential nursing care

See text pages
_____

IV. Psychologic influences on sexual response: gender identity and sex role; knowledge; emotions (e.g., love, anger, guilt); fantasies; expectations; religious, family, and ethnic beliefs

See text pages
_____

V. Essential nursing care

A. Nursing assessment
1. Assess personal belief system on sexuality and how that may impact on communicating with clients about sexual health.
2. Obtain sexual and menstrual history.
3. Assess client's level of knowledge about reproduction and sexual function.
4. Determine client's attitudes, beliefs, and feelings about sexual expression.
5. Identify any problems in the client's sexual activity.
6. Identify any menstrual disorders.

B. Nursing diagnoses
1. Knowledge deficit related to reproduction, menstruation, or sexual response
2. Sexual dysfunction and/or altered sexuality patterns related to dyspareunia
3. Anxiety or fear related to sexual practices and expectations
4. Self-esteem disturbance related to sexual functioning
5. Alteration in lifestyle related to symptomology of PMS

C. Nursing intervention
1. Teach couple about anatomy and physiology of reproduction and sexual response.
2. Teach about the range of influences on individual sexual expression and practices.
3. Refer for evaluation of dyspareunia.
4. Reassure couple about diversity of normal sexual function.
5. Provide emotional support and reassurance.
6. Encourage communication between sexual partners.
7. Refer for evaluation of menstrual disorder.

D. Nursing evaluation
1. Couple understand the specifics of reproduction and sexual response.
2. Couple have decreased fear and anxiety about sexual practices.
3. Couple have enhanced communication about sexual relationship.
4. Dyspareunia or menstrual disorder has been evaluated and treated.

1. Which of the following female structures secretes mucus that enhances the viability and mobility of sperm deposited in the vagina?
   a. Montgomery's tubercles
   b. Sertoli cells
   c. Leydig's cells
   d. Bartholin's glands

2. In the male, spermatogenesis occurs in the:
   a. Vas deferens.
   b. Prostate gland.
   c. Epididymis.
   d. Testes.

3. In which of the following situations would spermatogenesis be most affected?
   a. Impotence
   b. Vasectomy
   c. Undescended testes
   d. Prostatectomy

4. Estrogen levels are highest during which phase of the menstrual cycle?
   a. Menstrual
   b. Proliferative
   c. Secretory
   d. Ischemic

5. Measurements of the female pelvis are done to:
   a. Evaluate the proper fitting of a diaphragm.
   b. Assess the likelihood of becoming pregnant.
   c. Determine the ability to have a vaginal birth.
   d. Predict the gestational age of the fetus.

6. Marjorie, age 18, is discussing her recurring dysmenorrhea with the clinic nurse. Appropriate self-care measures to teach Marjorie include:
   a. Taking ibuprofen twice a day throughout the menstrual cycle.
   b. Maintaining a regular exercise program.
   c. Increasing fluid intake to 6–8 glasses of water a day.
   d. Applying cold packs to lower abdomen.

7. Kelly, age 50, asks the nurse if she still needs to use her diaphragm since she has not had a menstrual period during the past 8 months. The best response for the nurse is:
   a. "Do you think you might be pregnant?"
   b. "It appears you are in menopause now, and you do not need to use birth control measures any longer."
   c. "You need to continue to use your diaphragm until you have had 12 consecutive months without a period."
   d. "As long as you aren't having hot flashes, you are not menopausal."

8. Phyllis, age 22 and newly married, is discussing her sexual concerns with the nurse. She states, "I don't understand why my husband can have only 1 orgasm. It's so frustrating for me." The first nursing action should be to:
   a. Collect more data about the problem.
   b. Provide sexual information.
   c. Set up a counseling program.
   d. Refer the client to a sex therapist.

9. While discussing the human sexual response cycle with Phyllis, the nurse reviews the phases with Phyllis. The correct order of the sexual response cycle is:
   a. Excitement, orgasm, plateau, and resolution.
   b. Excitement, plateau, orgasm, and resolution.
   c. Resolution, excitement, plateau, and orgasm.
   d. Resolution, plateau, orgasm, and excitement.

10. Alma experiences excessive menstrual flow. She says to the nurse, "I feel so tired and generally sluggish even after the bleeding stops." The nurse understands that nutritional intake of iron-rich food is important. She suggests that Alma increase her intake of:

   a. Milk.
   b. Orange juice.
   c. Carrots.
   d. Dark-green leafy vegetables.

11. The school nurse is discussing menstruation with a group of 11-year-old girls. One girl asks the nurse, "Will everyone know when I have my period?" The nurse's best response is:

   a. "No, not unless you tell them."
   b. "You might think everyone knows, but no one but you knows what is happening to your body."
   c. "Sometimes, too many trips to the bathroom make people suspicious."
   d. "You should talk with your mom to see how she handled this."

12. Roseanne is being evaluated for premenstrual syndrome (PMS). Which of the following symptoms are commonly identified with PMS?

   a. Headaches, fluid retention, and irritability
   b. Fever, headaches, and skin rashes
   c. Hot flashes, dizziness, and palpitations
   d. Dyspareunia, dysuria, and fatigue

ANSWERS

1. Correct answer is d. The Bartholin's glands are located in the vaginal opening and secrete a mucus that enhances sperm viability.

   a. Montgomery's tubercles are small papillae located in the nipple area of the breast.
   b. Sertoli cells are located in the male testes and function in nourishment and protection of developing sperm.
   c. Leydig's cells are located in the testes and produce testosterone.

2. Correct answer is d. Sperm are formed and stored in the testes.

   a. The vas deferens is a duct that allows sperm to travel from the ejaculatory duct of the epididymis to the urethra.
   b. The prostate gland secretes fluid and nutrients for the sperm.
   c. The epididymis is a reservoir for sperm.

3. Correct answer is c. Spermatogenesis is a heat-sensitive process. If the testes remain abdominally located, the temperature can be 2°–3° higher than the scrotal temperature. This can greatly interfere with sperm production.

   a. Impotence is the inability of the male to achieve or maintain an erection. There is no relationship to spermatogenesis.
   b. After a vasectomy, spermatogenesis continues to proceed. However, the pathway from testes to urethra is interrupted.
   d. Spermatogenesis occurs in the testes; removal of the prostate gland does not impair sperm production.

4. Correct answer is b. Estrogen levels rise sharply just before ovulation during the proliferative phase (days 6–14).

   a. During the menstrual phase (days 1–5), estrogen levels are low.
   c. There is a rapid decline in estrogen during the secretory phase (days 15–26), and progesterone levels increase.
   d. Both estrogen and progesterone levels decrease during the ischemic phase (days 27–28) in response to the degeneration of the corpus luteum.

5. Correct answer is c. Measurements of the pelvis include diameters of the inlet, midpelvis, and outlet, and determine the ability of the fetus to pass from uterus through birth canal.

   a. There is no need to measure the pelvis for diaphragm fitting. Rather, the diaphragm size is related to the size of the anterior vaginal wall and cervix.

b. Ability to achieve pregnancy does not relate to the size of the pelvis.

d. There is no relationship between size of fetus and size of pelvis in terms of gestational age.

6. **Correct answer is b.** Exercise increases sense of well-being as well as preventing muscle spasms that occur with dysmenorrhea.

   a. Prostaglandin inhibitors such as ibuprofen are beneficial for pain relief. However, taking them throughout menstrual cycle is not warranted.
   c. Normal fluid intake should be 6–8 glasses of water a day. This has no direct effect on dysmenorrhea.
   d. Cold packs are inappropriate. A heating pad or a warm tub bath or shower may be beneficial since heat increases blood supply and, as a result, decreases muscle spasms.

7. **Correct answer is c.** Menopause is not clearly present until 12 consecutive months of no menses.

   a. This is an inappropriate response given age of client, the fact that she has been using a diaphragm, and the fact that it has been 8 months since the last menstrual period.
   b. This response is inappropriate and gives misinformation to the client; Kelly may still ovulate periodically.
   d. Not all menopausal women experience hot flashes.

8. **Correct answer is a.** Further assessment to obtain more information regarding Phyllis's understanding of the normal male sexual response is needed.

   b. Once the nurse knows Phyllis's level of understanding of the sexual response, she can provide teaching.
   c and d. The nurse does not have enough information to warrant either a counseling program or a referral to a sex therapist.

9. **Correct answer is b.** The sexual response cycle consists of excitement, or foreplay, followed by a plateau with engorgement of vagina and labia and clitoral retraction in the female and elevation of testes and distension of urethra with semen in the male. This is followed by orgasm, or climax, when there are contractions of clitoris, vagina, and uterus and contraction of penis and ejaculation of semen. Resolution, the final stage, is relaxation and a return to an unaroused state.

   a, c, and **d.** These responses are incorrect.

10. **Correct answer is d.** Eating dark-green leafy vegetables that are rich in vitamin C and iron often enhances absorption of iron.

    a. Milk is a poor source of iron.
    b. Orange juice is rich in vitamin C but poor in iron.
    c. Carrots are very low in iron but a good source of vitamin A.

11. **Correct answer is b.** The nurse understands that 11-year-old girls still are cognitively immature and may have "marginal thinking." Her response needs to be truthful as well as disperse any false ideas.

    a. Although a correct statement, it does not address the girl's uncertainty or insecurity.
    c. This is an inappropriate response that could cause the girl increased anxiety.
    d. Although this is a good suggestion that the nurse could add to her response, it does not answer the girl's question.

12. **Correct answer is a.** PMS includes cyclic recurrent symptoms such as irritability, fluid retention, headaches, nervousness, and food cravings.

    b. A fever should not be seen in PMS. This would indicate viral or bacterial influence on the body.
    c. This group of symptoms is not generally seen in PMS but rather in menopause.
    d. Dyspareunia (painful intercourse) and dysuria (painful urination) are not common symptoms of PMS.

3

Genetics, Conception, and Embryonic and Fetal Development

NURSING HIGHLIGHTS

1. To provide essential prenatal nursing care to pregnant clients and their families, nurse should understand the process of fertilization, the normal development process of embryo and fetus from conception to birth, and the functioning of intrauterine systems.
2. Ovum is fertile for 24 hours after ovulation; sperm is capable of fertilizing for 24–48 hours after being deposited in female.

3. Fetus is at greatest risk from teratogens during embryonic stage of development. Nurse should know substances that are harmful to fetus.
4. Fetal and maternal blood supplies are completely separate, breached only by a defect in placental membrane.

GLOSSARY

centromere—portion of chromosome where chromatids join
chromatid—filaments that make up chromosome and separate at cell division
decidua—endometrium of pregnancy that allows for zygote implantation
diploid—having 2 sets of chromosomes, as in somatic cells
fertilization—fusion of sperm and ovum
gamete—mature sex cell (ovum and spermatozoon)
haploid—having single set of chromosomes, as in gametes
heterozygous—having 2 dissimilar genes at the same site on paired chromosomes
homozygous—having 2 similar genes at the same site on paired chromosomes
karyotype—chromosomal constitution of nucleus of the cell
teratogen—factor producing structural or functional defects in developing embryo

ENHANCED OUTLINE

I. Basic genetic components of humans

A. Chromosomes: structures in the nucleus of somatic cells that transmit genetic information

> See text pages
> _____

1. Chromosomes are composed of linear strands of DNA (deoxyribonucleic acid) and protein.
2. There are 46 (23 pairs) chromosomes in each cell.
   a) 22 pairs of autosomes (somatic cells)
   b) 1 pair of sex chromosomes: either XX (female) or XY (male)
3. Each chromosome contains two halves, called chromatids, which are joined at a location called a centromere.
4. Chromosomes are classified according to length and the position of the centromere.

B. DNA
1. Each DNA strand splits to form ribonucleic acid (RNA).
2. RNA passes out of nucleus to carry genetic code to cytoplasm of cell.

C. Genes: biologic unit of heredity
1. Genes have definite positions on DNA strands, arranged in linear order.

2. Genes contain coded information for individual characteristics of offspring.
3. Each half of each pair of chromosomes contains genes that are either homozygous or heterozygous.

II. Processes of cell reproduction

See text pages
_____

A. Mitosis: process of somatic cell division that is responsible for growth and development of all humans; allows body cells to replace themselves throughout a person's life
   1. The 2 cells formed by division of parent cell contain the same number of chromosomes as parent cell: diploid number of 46.
   2. Genetic components of each new cell are the same as those of parent cell.

B. Meiosis: process of 2 successive cell divisions that produces female ova and male spermatozoa
   1. The process of development of ova and spermatozoa is called gametogenesis.
      a) Oogenesis (formation of mature ova): First meiotic division begins before birth in ovary of fetus, is arrested until puberty, and is completed while ovum is in ovarian follicle; second meiotic division begins at ovulation and is completed when penetrated by sperm.
      b) Spermatogenesis (formation of mature sperm): Both meiotic divisions occur in the testes during puberty; sperm mature when discharged in ejaculate.
   2. Each gamete has half the number of chromosomes (haploid number of 23) of the original cell: 1 chromosome from each pair of autosomal chromosomes in parent cell and 1 sex chromosome.
   3. Chromosomal abnormalities can occur during the second division if an extra chromosome is formed or if chromosomes break. (See Chapter 4, section II,A, for a discussion of chromosomal abnormalities.)

C. Sex determination: established at time of fertilization by the male sex chromosome
   1. Mature ovum is always X type.
   2. Mature spermatozoon is either X or Y type.
   3. Female is produced if spermatozoon contains X type; male is produced if sperm contains Y type.

III. Fertilization and implantation

See text pages

A. Prefertilization activities
  1. Ovum moves to outer third (ampulla) of fallopian tube, under influence of estrogen.
  2. Sperm undergoes changes prior to fertilization.
     a) Capacitation: removal of sperm's protective coat
     b) Acrosome reaction: loss of membrane to allow attachment to ovum

B. Conception
  1. When 1 sperm fuses to ovum through ovum's 2 outer layers (zona pellucida and corona radiata), no other sperm can enter.
  2. New cell (zygote) forms, containing 46 chromosomes; mitotic cell division begins.

C. Implantation (nidation)
  1. Zygote undergoes rapid mitotic development (cleavage) while traveling down fallopian tube.
     a) Initial division results in 2 cells called blastomeres.
     b) Over 3–4 days, 16 blastomeres develop, forming ball-like cellular structure (morula).

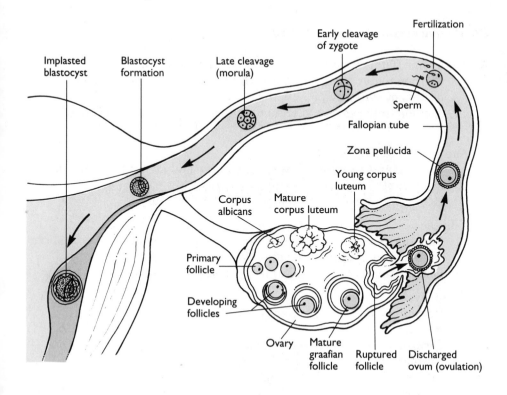

Figure 3-1
Fertilization Process

2. Morula is delivered to uterus.
3. Cavity develops within cell mass.
   a) Inner solid cell mass (blastocyst) becomes the embryo and amnion.
   b) Outer cell-feeding layer (trophoblast) becomes chorion that is responsible for embedding ovum.
4. Trophoblast attaches to uterine wall.
5. Blastocyst implants completely in uterine wall within 7–10 days of fertilization.
6. Uterine lining (endometrium) thickens to allow implantation and nourishment of ovum.

D. Multiple pregnancies: Twins occur in 1 of 90 births.
   1. Dizygotic (fraternal): fertilization of 2 ova by 2 sperm; genetically distinct; same or different sexes
   2. Monozygotic (identical): division of inner cell mass into 2 parts at blastocyst stage; genetically similar and same sex

IV. Prenatal developmental structures

See text pages
_____

A. Embryonic (fetal) membranes: protect and support embryo
   1. Chorion (outer layer, covered with chorionic villi): becomes fetal portion of placenta
   2. Amnion (inner layer): surrounds embryo and yolk sac and contains fluid

B. Amniotic fluid (bag of waters)
   1. Protects and cushions developing embryo and allows freedom of fetal movement
   2. Helps maintain an even temperature for the fetus

C. Yolk sac
   1. Functions only in early embryonic life to provide nutrients to embryo while uteroplacental circulation is being established
   2. Forms primitive red blood cells until embryonic hemopoiesis begins

D. Germ layers
   1. Responsible for development of all tissues, organs, and organ systems
   2. Formed when blastocysts differentiate 10–14 days after conception
   3. Develop into different body parts
      a) Ectoderm (outer layer): epidermis, epidermal tissue, nervous system, external sense organs, mucous membranes of mouth and anus

b) Mesoderm (middle layer): connective tissue, bone, cartilage, muscle, blood and blood vessels, kidneys, lymphatics, gonads, pericardium, peritoneum

c) Endoderm (inner layer): respiratory and digestive tracts, bladder, urethra

V. Fetal development

See text pages

A. Ways to determine length of pregnancy
   1. 40 weeks (280 days) from beginning of last menstrual period (LMP) to birth
   2. 38 weeks (266 days) from fertilization; more accurate to measure from time of conception

B. Stages of prenatal development
   1. Preembryonic stage: days 1–14, beginning at conception
      a) Rapid cellular multiplication and differentiation
      b) Formation of embryonic membranes and germ layers
      c) Possibility of poor implantation and spontaneous abortion due to exposure to teratogens
   2. Embryonic stage: day 15 until 8 weeks
      a) Differentiation of tissues into organs
      b) Development of external features
      c) Embryo most vulnerable to effects of teratogens, such as viruses, drugs, radiation, and infection
         (1) Results in major congenital abnormalities
         (2) Causes either necrosis or biochemical paralysis of the developing cells
   3. Fetal stage: week 9 to birth
      a) Refinement and perfection of each organ system and external features occur; weight increases from about 14 g at week 9 to 3000–3600 g at term.
         (1) 9–12 weeks: Head is prominent as brain develops; fetal heartbeats are heard by Doppler device.
         (2) 13–16 weeks: Skeleton ossifies and muscles mature; fetus makes sucking motions; sex can be easily determined.
         (3) 17–20 weeks: Mother feels movement (quickening); heartbeat can be heard with fetoscope; fetus has regular schedule of movement; hair on head, eyebrows, and eyelashes are present; lanugo (fine, downy hair) covers whole body.
         (4) 21–24 weeks: Fetal movement increases; fetal respiratory movements begin; skin is wrinkled; fetus has grasping and startle reflexes.
         (5) 25–28 weeks: Eyes open; circulatory and respiratory systems have developed; fetus can breathe, but lungs are not fully matured; nervous system starts to regulate body functions; fetus has a chance to survive outside womb.

       (6) 29–32 weeks: Muscle and fat increase.

       (7) 33–36 weeks: Skin becomes less wrinkled; subcutaneous fat develops; lanugo starts to disappear; nails reach fingertips; surfactant system of lungs matures at about 36 weeks.

       (8) 37 weeks–term: Fetus is full-term at 38 weeks; lanugo disappears; vernix caseosa increases.

    b) Fetus is less vulnerable to teratogens, which may, however, cause physiologic defects or minor morphologic abnormalities.

VI. Intrauterine systems

See text pages

A. Placenta

    1. Anatomy: connected to fetus by umbilical cord

       a) Maternal portion consists of decidua basalis.

       b) Fetal portion consists of chorionic villi.

    2. Development: begins after third week of gestation

       a) Trophoblast cells of chorionic villi form spaces in maternal tissue; intervillous spaces fill with maternal blood; fetal villi grow into spaces.

       b) Connective tissue layer of chorionic villi develops into 15–20 segments (cotyledons), forming maternal surface of placenta.

       c) Branching villi within each cotyledon form a complex vascular system for exchange of gases and nutrients.

       d) Fetal and maternal circulations are separated by tissue layers.

    3. Functions: communication between maternal and fetal circulations

       a) Transfers gases, nutrients, maternal antibodies, and wastes

       b) Produces hormones

       c) Detoxifies some drugs and chemicals

    4. Mechanisms of transmission

       a) Simple diffusion: transport of gases that depends on partial pressure of each gas (e.g., oxygen, carbon dioxide)

       b) Facilitated diffusion: transport of substances that are in a concentration greater on maternal than on fetal side (e.g., glucose)

       c) Active transport: movement of substances against concentration gradient that requires energy expenditure by cells (e.g., amino acids and water-soluble vitamins)

       d) Bulk flow: transfer of substances against hydrostatic or osmotic gradient by passage through membrane micropores (e.g., water and dissolved electrolytes)

       e) Pinocytosis: transfer of particles (e.g., albumin and immunoglobulin) by engulfing them

5. Factors affecting transfer: size of molecule, electrical charge, rate of blood flow, placental mass, blood saturation, lipid solubility
   a) Defects or breaks in membrane allow fetal red blood cells to leak to maternal circulation, causing sensitization of Rh-negative mother to Rh-positive fetus.
   b) Harmful substances (viruses, bacteria, drugs) can pass from mother to fetus.
6. Placental hormones
   a) Human chorionic gonadotropin (hCG): prevents normal involution of corpus luteum at end of menstrual cycle; thought to be responsible for nausea and vomiting of early pregnancy
   b) Progesterone: enables provision of nutrients, develops uterine lining for implantation, maintains endometrium, and decreases uterine contractility
   c) Estrogen: causes enlargement of uterus and breasts and develops breast ductal system for lactation
   d) Human placental lactogen (hPL): ensures maternal provision of protein, glucose, and minerals to fetus
   e) Prostaglandins: found in high concentrations in the amnion, chorion, and decidua; thought to play a role in labor (specific function not yet understood)
   f) Relaxin: thought to relax the symphysis pubis and other pelvic joints and to soften cervix; may be produced by placenta

B. Umbilical cord: links embryo and fetus to placenta
   1. Contains 2 umbilical arteries and 1 umbilical vein
   2. Wharton's jelly: surrounds umbilical vessels in cord to prevent compression

C. Fetal circulation
   1. Provides oxygen and nutrients to fetus and carries carbon dioxide and wastes from fetus
      a) Oxygenated maternal blood leaves placenta, entering fetus through fetal (umbilical) vein.
      b) Special vessels direct fetal blood flow.
         (1) Ductus venosus carries blood from umbilical vein to inferior vena cava, bypassing liver, which gets a part of oxygenated blood directly from vein.
         (2) Foramen ovale allows blood to flow directly from right atrium into left atrium, to left ventricle, and into ascending aorta.
         (3) Ductus arteriosus carries blood from pulmonary artery, into descending aorta, bypassing lungs.
      c) Deoxygenated fetal blood returns to placenta through umbilical arteries.

2. Provides different concentrations of oxygen
   a) Highest to head, neck, brain, heart, and upper limbs
   b) Lesser to abdominal organs and lower body
   c) Responsible for cephalocaudal (head-to-tail) fetal development

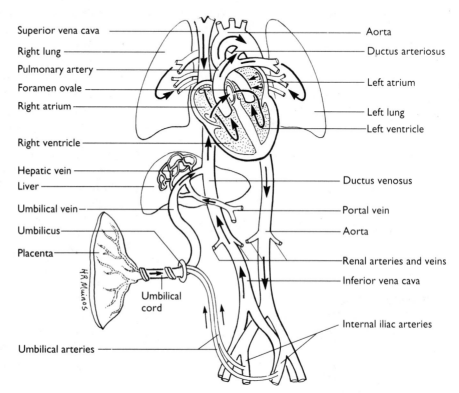

Figure 3-2
Fetal Circulation

1. The phase of cellular division during which the number of chromosomes in oocytes and in spermatocytes is reduced by one-half is called:

    a. Mitosis.
    b. Miosis.
    c. Meiosis.
    d. Gametogenesis.

2. Fusion of sperm and ovum forms a:

    a. Zygote.
    b. Blastomere.
    c. Morula.
    d. Gamete.

3. The sex of offspring is determined at the time of:

    a. Meiosis.
    b. Fertilization.
    c. Capacitation.
    d. Oogenesis.

4. Fertilization of the ovum occurs most often in the:

    a. Uterine endometrium.
    b. Ovary.
    c. Cervix.
    d. Fallopian tube.

5. A characteristic of dizygotic, or fraternal, twins is that they:

    a. Have the same genetic complement.
    b. Are always male.
    c. Share the same placenta.
    d. Develop from 2 ova.

6. Ashley, gravida 2 para 1, is being seen in the prenatal clinic for her initial assessment. She tells the nurse that she just felt the baby move for the first time this week. Based on this information, the nurse estimates Ashley's baby to be approximately:

    a. 12 weeks.
    b. 16 weeks.
    c. 20 weeks.
    d. 24 weeks.

7. Ashley tells the nurse that the first day of her last menstrual period was September 1. Ashley also states that she had some slight vaginal bleeding later in September. She asks the nurse, "Is this normal? Could something have happened to my baby?" The nurse's best response is:

    a. "This sometimes occurs as the fertilized egg attaches to the uterus and is normal."
    b. "You will need to have further tests to see if anything happened to your baby."
    c. "That probably was a miscarriage of a twin."
    d. "It's nothing to worry about."

8. As Ashley's initial prenatal visit continues, she informs the nurse that she had "the flu" at the end of September. The nurse understands that effects of teratogens are most harmful to fetal organ development during the:

    a. Preconception stage.
    b. Preembryonic stage.
    c. Embryonic stage.
    d. Fetal stage.

9. The role of the placental hormone human chorionic gonadotropin (hCG) is to:

    a. Develop the uterine lining for implantation.
    b. Develop breast duct system for lactation.
    c. Regulate maternal metabolism to supply nutrients to the fetus.
    d. Prevent the normal involution of the corpus luteum.

10. The transfer of maternal estrogen to the fetus is seen in the newborn as:

    a. Soft skin.
    b. Cheesy vernix.
    c. Enlarged breast tissue in both boys and girls.
    d. Presence of subcutaneous fat.

11. Oxygen is transported to the fetus via the placenta. The mechanism by which this occurs is called:

    a. Active transport.
    b. Hydrostatic pressure.
    c. Diffusion.
    d. Pinocytosis.

12. With the clamping of the umbilical cord at birth, large amounts of blood are returned to the newborn's heart and lungs, causing equal pressure in the left atrium and right atrium. This pressure causes the closure of:

    a. Ductus arteriosus.
    b. Ductus venosus.
    c. Umbilical arteries.
    d. Foramen ovale.

ANSWERS

1. **Correct answer is c.** Meiosis is the process of cell division during the formation of gametes that results in cells having a haploid number of chromosomes.

   a. Mitosis is the ordinary process of cell division that results in the formation of 2 daughter cells. Each daughter cell receives identical diploid complements of chromosomes.
   b. Miosis is excessive contraction of the pupil.
   d. Gametogenesis is the development of the male and female sex cells (gametes).

2. **Correct answer is a.** A zygote is the cell resulting from the union of a male and a female gamete and containing 46 chromosomes.

   b. Once the zygote enters the rapid mitotic division called cleavage, it divides into many cells called blastomeres.
   c. A morula is a solid mass of cells (blastomeres) formed by cleavage.
   d. A gamete is 1 of 2 haploid reproductive cells whose union is necessary in sexual reproduction to initiate the development of a new individual.

3. **Correct answer is b.** At the time of fertilization, the sex of the offspring is determined by the combination of the spermatozoon (either X or Y) and the ovum (X). XX becomes female; XY becomes male.

   a. Meiosis is the process of 2 successive cell divisions that produce female ova and male spermatozoa.
   c. Capacitation is the removal of the sperm's protective coat.
   d. Oogenesis is the maturation process of an ovum.

4. **Correct answer is d.** Fertilization takes place in the ampulla of the fallopian tube. High estrogen levels during ovulation increase the contractility of the fallopian tubes, which aids the movement of the ovum down the tube.

   a. Implantation and attachment of the fertilized egg occur most often in the upper part of the posterior uterine walls.
   b. The ovaries release the ovum during ovulation.
   c. The cervix is the lower portion of the uterus extending into the vagina.

5. **Correct answer is d.** Dizygotic twins are the result of the maturation of 2 ova during 1 ovulation cycle, which are fertilized at the same time or within hours.

   a. This is a characteristic of monozygotic, or identical, twins. Dizygotic twins have genetic makeup no more similar than siblings born at different times.
   b. Dizygotic twins can be of different sexes or the same sex.
   c. Dizygotic twins have separate placentas.

6. **Correct answer is c.** Quickening, or maternal identification of fetal movement, occurs at approximately 20 weeks' gestation.

   a and b. At 12–16 weeks, the nurse could hear fetal heart tones with a Doppler device. It is unlikely at these stages to have the mother identify fetal movement.
   d. At 24 weeks, the client would feel fetal movements but not for the first time.

7. **Correct answer is a.** This is called implantation bleeding and sometimes occurs as the trophoblast burrows into the uterine endometrium. This response provides information and answers Ashley's question.

   b. This is an inappropriate response since it could lead Ashley to think something is wrong with the fetus.
   c. A single twin cannot be discharged.
   d. This is an inappropriate response; it minimizes Ashley's concerns and does not provide a clear explanation of why the occurrence should not be a source of concern.

8. **Correct answer is c.** During the embryonic state, initial development of tissues into organs occurs. Exposure to viruses, drugs, radiation, and infections during this time may result in congenital abnormalities.

   a. Teratogens to which the client is exposed prior to conception may have an effect on her health but do not harm a future fetus.
   b. The preembryonic stage is the beginning stage of conception. During this time, exposure to teratogens may lead to poor implantation and spontaneous abortion.
   d. During the fetal stage, physiologic defects or minor morphologic abnormalities may result from exposure.

9. **Correct answer is d.** The hormone hCG prevents the normal involution of the corpus luteum at the end of the menstrual cycle. If the corpus luteum stops functioning before the 11th week of pregnancy, spontaneous abortion occurs.

   a. Progesterone develops the uterine lining for implantation, maintains the endometrium, and decreases uterine contractility.
   b. Estrogen functions to develop breast duct system for lactation.
   c. Human placental lactogen (hPL) ensures the fetus of nutrients from the mother via facilitated diffusion.

10. **Correct answer is c.** Because maternal estrogen is transmitted to the fetus, it is not uncommon to see enlarged breast tissue in both boys and girls during the first few days of life.

    a, b, and **d.** All are signs of a well-developed full-term newborn but do not relate to maternal estrogen levels.

11. **Correct answer is c.** Oxygen is transported via simple diffusion: substances move from an area of higher concentration to an area of lower concentration.

    a. Active transport provides movement of substances against a concentration gradient and requires energy by cells. This is how amino acids and glucose are transferred across the placenta.
    b. Hydrostatic pressure allows the bulk flow of water by passage through membrane micropores.
    d. Pinocytosis is a method of transferring large particles (i.e., immunoglobulins) by engulfing them.

12. **Correct answer is d.** The equal pressure in the left atrium and right atrium causes the closure of the foramen ovale. It remains closed and eventually disappears. This converts fetal circulation into newborn circulation.

    a and **b.** With closure of the foramen ovale, the ductus arteriosus and ductus venosus no longer need to shunt blood. Both are eventually converted into ligaments.
    c. After birth, the umbilical arteries fill with clotted blood and are eventually converted to abdominal ligaments.

4

Special Reproductive Issues

NURSING HIGHLIGHTS

1. Nurse should be aware that in-depth fertility diagnosis and treatment are time-consuming, expensive, and stressful and may strain a couple's relationship.
2. Timing of infertility tests within the menstrual and ovulation cycle is often critical to securing accurate results.
3. Nurse should not exhibit reluctance or embarrassment when discussing infertile couple's sexual history and habits but should convey empathy and understanding.
4. Nurse should remain objective, supporting a couple's decision about continuing or terminating a pregnancy after diagnosis of genetic abnormality.

5. Nurse should participate in care of abortion clients only if certain that personal and moral beliefs do not conflict with abortion.
6. Nurse should explain all aspects of contraceptive methods, including accurate effectiveness rates and risks, so client or couple can choose most appropriate method.

GLOSSARY

anovulation—failure of ovaries to produce, mature, or release eggs

dermatoglyphics—study of ridge patterns on skin, particularly on hands and feet, used in genetic evaluations

endometrial biopsy—procedure during which a sample of the endometrium is taken from the uterus to examine for dysfunction of the luteal phase of the menstrual cycle

gamete intrafallopian transfer (GIFT)—human fertilization technique in which ova are retrieved from the woman and injected into her fallopian tubes along with the man's sperm for fertilization in the woman's body

hysterosalpingography—procedure producing x-rays of uterus and fallopian tubes to detect abnormalities

hysteroscopy—visual examination of cervical canal and uterine cavity with an endoscope

in vitro fertilization—human fertilization technique in which ova are fertilized with sperm in a laboratory and then injected into the uterus

karyotype—chromosome makeup of a human cell; microphotograph showing the chromosome arrangement of an individual

nondisjunction—unequal distribution of chromosomes during cell reproduction

zygote intrafallopian transfer (ZIFT)—human fertilization technique in which ova are fertilized with sperm in a laboratory and transferred to the fallopian tubes

ENHANCED OUTLINE

I. Infertility

A. Definition: inability to conceive after a period of unprotected intercourse or inability to carry a fetus to live birth

B. Types
   1. Primary: never pregnant
   2. Secondary: pregnant at least once; now unable to conceive or sustain pregnancy
   3. Sterility: conception not possible, with irremediable cause

C. Criteria for initiating fertility evaluation
   1. 1 year unprotected intercourse without conception
   2. For couples over 30, 6 months of unprotected intercourse without conception

See text pages

D. Causes of infertility
   1. Female
      a) Cervical mucus that is incompatible with sperm: due to infection, immunologic response, or antisperm antibodies
      b) Obstruction between cervix and fallopian tubes: due to fibroid tumors, polyps, adhesions, endometritis, or endometriosis
      c) Tubal problems: due to adhesions, pelvic inflammatory disease (PID), endometriosis, tubal ligation, or ectopic pregnancy
      d) Ovarian problems
         (1) Anovulation: due to endocrine disorders, disease, infection, cysts, medications, or low body-fat ratio due to diet or exercise
         (2) Obstruction between ovary and fimbria: due to adhesions, endometriosis, or PID
      e) Failure of endometrium to allow implantation and normal growth of embryo and fetus: due to anovulation, infection, or luteal phase defect
   2. Male
      a) Low sperm count (<20 million/ml) or insufficient motility (<50% mobile after 2 hours): due to varicocele, medications, infections, postpuberty mumps, exposure to toxic chemicals or radiation, substance abuse, or excess heat to scrotal area
      b) Abnormal reproductive tract secretions: due to infection, tumors, or autoimmunity to semen
      c) Testicular disease
      d) Obstruction of reproductive tract: due to infection, vasectomy, or tumors
      e) Inability to deposit sperm within female vagina so that it reaches cervix: due to premature ejaculation, hypospadias, or erectile problems

E. Assessment of female infertility
   1. Comprehensive history
      a) Fertility: duration of impaired fertility, type and length of contraception, time without contraception, previous tests and treatment
      b) Obstetric: number of pregnancies, number of abortions, time required to become pregnant, complications of pregnancy, duration of lactation
      c) Menstrual: menarche; frequency, length, and abnormalities of cycle; pain
      d) Medical: chronic or hereditary disease, infections, medications

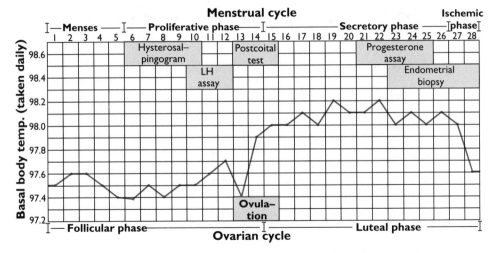

Figure 4-1
Timing of Fertility Tests During Menstrual and Ovarian Cycles

    e) Sexual: libido, dyspareunia, history of sexual abuse, techniques for and timing and frequency of intercourse

    f) Surgical: pelvic or abdominal procedures

    g) Lifestyle: occupational and environmental exposures; diet; use of alcohol, tobacco, or drugs; exercise patterns

    h) Psychosocial: motivation for wanting children, status of relationship with partner, religious and cultural considerations, pressure from family and friends

2. Physical examination

    a) General health and nutritional status, including endocrine evaluation

    b) Reproductive tract: pelvic, bimanual, rectovaginal examinations

3. Laboratory studies

    a) Complete blood count (CBC), urinalysis (U/A), serology, Pap smear, Rh factor and blood grouping

    b) Endocrine studies: thyroid function tests and glucose tolerance tests

    c) Other lab tests as needed

4. Diagnostic tests

    a) Tests to detect ovulatory dysfunction

        (1) Basal body temperature (BBT) recording: to help identify follicular and luteal phase abnormalities and to determine best times to have intercourse

        (2) Hormone assays

            (a) Serum or urine luteinizing hormone (LH) assay: to determine day of LH surge (day of maximum fertility); testing done daily right before expected ovulation

            (b) Serum progesterone assay: to determine ovulation and corpus luteum function; done during luteal phase

           (3) Endometrial biopsy: to determine ovulation and presence and adequacy of secretory tissues; done during luteal phase

           (4) Ultrasound: to determine follicular changes

        b) Cervical mucus tests: to determine whether cervical mucus is receptive to sperm

        c) Postcoital test: to evaluate interaction of cervical mucus and sperm; done during ovulation

        d) Tubal patency tests (hysterosalpingography, hysteroscopy, laparoscopy, culdoscopy)

  F. Assessment of male infertility

    1. Comprehensive history

        a) Surgical: herniorrhaphy, vasectomy, local injuries to scrotal area

        b) Medical: chronic diseases, infections, postpuberty mumps, varicocele, medications

        c) Personal: age, type of underwear (constrictive garments), bathing habits (hot baths)

        d) Fertility: previous fathering with different sexual partner

        e) Sexual: libido, erectile problems, techniques for and timing and frequency of intercourse

        f) Lifestyle: occupational and environmental exposures, especially irradiation exposures; diet; use of alcohol, tobacco, or drugs

        g) Psychosocial: same as section I,E,1,h of this chapter

    2. Physical examination

        a) General health and endocrine status

        b) Urologic examination

        c) Rectal examination

    3. Laboratory evaluation: CBC, U/A, serology, Rh factor and blood grouping

    4. Diagnostic tests

        a) Semen analysis to evaluate sperm production, motility, and viability (see Client Teaching Checklist, "Collecting Usable Semen Sample")

        b) Postcoital test (same as section I,E,4,c of this chapter)

        c) Sperm antibody tests

  G. Management of infertility

    1. Maximizing timing and frequency of intercourse

    2. Medications: hormones and fertility agents

        a) Clomiphene citrate and human menopausal gonadotropin: to induce ovulation

        b) Guaifenesin and doxycycline: to improve cervical mucus characteristics

    3. Surgery

Collecting Usable Semen Sample

Explanation to client:

✔ Specimen should be collected after abstaining from sex for several (2–3) days.
✔ Specimen may be collected by masturbation or by having intercourse.
✔ If specimen is collected during intercourse, special condom with no spermicidal agents must be used to catch sperm.
✔ Time of collection must be noted.
✔ Specimen should be carried to lab in a clean, dry glass or plastic container within 1–3 hours of collection.
✔ Specimen must be kept at body temperature during transport without use of artificial means (e.g., under arm).
✔ Final results are usually based on several test samples; 60–90 days must elapse between sperm collections.

4. Alternate means of conceiving or parenting: artificial insemination, in vitro fertilization (IVF), gamete intrafallopian transfer (GIFT), zygote intrafallopian transfer (ZIFT), adoption

H. Essential nursing care
   1. Nursing assessment
      a) Obtain comprehensive history (same as sections I,E,1 and I,F,1 of this chapter).
      b) Assess couple's knowledge of reproductive anatomy, physiology, and techniques.
      c) Observe interaction between couple.
   2. Nursing diagnoses
      a) Knowledge deficit related to:
         (1) Sexual anatomy or physiology
         (2) Sexual functioning
         (3) Tests and procedures
      b) Anxiety or fear related to condition and procedures
      c) Alteration in comfort related to testing procedures
      d) Situational low self-esteem related to inability to conceive
      e) Ineffective coping styles related to prolonged stress of infertility testing and/or failure to conceive
   3. Nursing intervention
      a) Provide educational information about testing procedures, treatments, and medications and the associated stress, time, and costs involved.
      b) Provide educational information about self-care measures and lifestyle changes that may enhance fertility (see Client Teaching Checklist, "Self-Care Actions to Enhance Fertility").

       c) Allay fears about tests and treatments; assist in testing and ordered treatments.

       d) Provide comfort measures during painful procedures.

       e) Help couple set realistic childbearing expectations.

       f) Help couple identify possible alternatives to childbearing.

       g) Help couple communicate with each other and with the health care team.

       h) Provide emotional support; be an empathetic listener.

       i) Refer couple for counseling or to support group if appropriate.

4. Nursing evaluation

       a) Couple understand procedures, tests, and alternatives to pregnancy.

       b) Couple demonstrate understanding of emotional, physical, and financial costs of fertility treatments.

       c) Couple are carrying out at-home procedures.

       d) Couple are aware of and have access to comfort measures during and after testing.

       e) Couple express decreased fear, embarrassment, or anxiety about infertility.

       f) Couple accept their situation and describe realistic expectations about outcome.

       g) Couple are able to begin resolving guilt, resentment, and anger.

✔ CLIENT TEACHING CHECKLIST ✔

Self-Care Actions to Enhance Fertility

Recommendations for client couple:

✔ Avoid petroleum-based vaginal lubricants and postcoital douches that could alter vaginal pH.

✔ Use the male superior position for sexual intercourse; after intercourse, the woman should elevate her hips and remain recumbent for 1 hour to help retain sperm.

✔ Have intercourse 1–3 times weekly, at intervals of at least 48 hours, to maximize fertilization potential.

✔ To increase sperm production, quality, and motility, the man should get adequate nutrition, reduce stress, wear loose-fitting underwear, avoid hot baths, and avoid recreational drugs.

II. Genetic disorders: diseases that are inherited or that result from chromosome reproduction defects (For review of genetics, see Chapter 3.)

See text pages
_____

A. Chromosomal abnormalities: can affect both autosomal (nonsex) and sex chromosomes; can be in number or in structure
   1. Conditions caused by autosomal chromosomes that are abnormal in number: often occur because of nondisjunction; often incompatible with life
      a) Trisomy: 1 gamete contains an extra chromosome. Trisomy 21 results in Down syndrome.
      b) Monosomy: 1 gamete has missing chromosome.
      c) Mosaicism: A zygote develops 2 different cell lines, each having a different chromosomal number.
   2. Conditions caused by autosomal chromosomes that are abnormal in structure
      a) Translocation: Chromosomes break and reconstruct in an abnormal arrangement.
      b) Additions or deletions of portions of chromosomes
   3. Sex chromosomal defects: deletion or addition of X chromosome (Turner's syndrome, Klinefelter's syndrome)

B. Single-gene disorders (inherited disorders)
   1. Autosomal dominant disorders: Only 1 member of a gene pair needs to be abnormal.
      a) With each pregnancy, affected parent has 50% chance of passing on abnormal gene.
      b) Both sexes are equally affected.
      c) Family history usually shows evidence of disorder in previous generations.
      d) Some disorders are polydactyly, Marfan's syndrome, Huntington's chorea, and neurofibromatosis.
      e) Individuals may be mildly or severely affected.
   2. Autosomal recessive disorders: Both members of 1 gene pair are abnormal.
      a) With each pregnancy, 2 parents who carry abnormal gene for a certain disorder have a 25% chance of having a child who manifests the disease.
      b) With each pregnancy, 2 parents who carry same abnormal gene have a 50% chance of having an offspring who is a carrier.
      c) Both sexes are affected.
      d) There is often no family history of the disease.
      e) Conditions are generally more severe and rarer than dominant-trait conditions.
      f) Presence of abnormal gene can sometimes be detected in carrier.
      g) Some disorders are cystic fibrosis, sickle cell anemia, Tay-Sachs disease, and phenylketonuria (PKU).

        3. Sex-linked (X-linked) recessive: X chromosome is abnormal.
- a) Disease almost always affects males (hemophilia).
- b) Affected males pass abnormal allele to all daughters, not to sons.
- c) When mothers are carriers, there is a 50% chance that each male offspring will have the disease and a 50% chance that each female offspring will be a carrier.

        4. Sex-linked dominant (rare); fragile-X syndrome (recently discovered)

C. Multifactorial disorders (e.g., spina bifida, club foot, cleft palate): have an inherited and an environmental component; increased risk of occurrence with each offspring

D. Prenatal screening and diagnostic procedures (see section IV of Chapter 6 for explanation of procedures)
1. Maternal serum alpha-fetoprotein (AFP) testing: preliminary screening done between 15th and 18th week of gestation; is not absolutely diagnostic (*must* be followed up if possible problem is noted)
2. Genetic ultrasound: done between 16th and 18th week of gestation
3. Genetic amniocentesis: done between 14th and 18th week of gestation
4. Chorionic villus sampling (CVS): alternative to amniocentesis; done earlier in the pregnancy (first trimester) with quicker results
5. Percutaneous umbilical blood sampling (PUBS): technique for obtaining blood from umbilical cord to provide quick diagnosis of chromosome abnormalities

E. Postnatal diagnostic procedures
1. Physical examination
2. Dermatoglyphic analysis
3. Lab tests: karyotyping; DNA analysis; blood tests to screen for inborn errors of metabolism, such as phenylketonuria (PKU), congenital hypothyroidism, galactosemia, maple syrup urine disease, and hemoglobinopathies

F. Essential nursing care during prenatal screening and testing and during genetic counseling
1. Take history; screen for risk factors (maternal age, maternal disease, family health history, reproductive history, ethnic background, environmental hazards).
2. Determine level of accurate knowledge about procedures (including risks to fetus); provide explanations as needed.
3. Encourage discussion between couple.
4. Make sure informed consent has been obtained.
5. Assist during testing.

6. Provide emotional support.
7. Assist couple through stages of depression and grieving if outcome of testing shows abnormality.
8. Refer at-risk family to counseling and support groups.

III. Abortion

See text pages
_____

A. Abortion procedures during first trimester
   1. Vacuum curettage
      a) After local anesthetic is applied to cervix, cervix is dilated, sometimes with laminaria (absorbent seaweed), and uterine lining is suctioned with cannula or curette and vacuum suction machine.
      b) Complications: infection, excessive bleeding, uterine blood clots, uterine or cervical trauma
   2. Dilation and curettage
      a) Cervix is dilated, and uterine endometrium is scraped out with a surgical curette.
      b) Complications: cervical trauma, uterine perforation, infection, bleeding
   3. Menstrual extraction
      a) Endometrium is aspirated with a cannula and syringe; done early in pregnancy (e.g., 2 weeks after missed period).
      b) Complications: hemorrhage, retained products, infection

B. Abortion procedures during second and third trimesters
   1. Dilation and extraction
      a) After cervical block or general anesthesia is administered, cervix is dilated with laminaria and contents of uterus are removed with suction and forceps.
      b) Complications: perforation of uterus, infection, excessive bleeding, retained products, cervical trauma, amniotic fluid embolism
   2. Hypertonic saline
      a) Hypertonic saline is instilled into amniotic cavity to induce uterine contractions and expulsion of fetus. Oxytocin may also be used.
      b) Complications: cervical trauma, uterine rupture, edema, renal failure, failed abortion, excessive bleeding, infection, tinnitus, headache, tachycardia, disseminated intravascular coagulation
   3. Hypertonic urea
      a) Hypertonic urea is injected using same procedure as used with hypertonic saline.
      b) Complications: high rate of failed abortion when not used with prostaglandins or oxytocin
   4. Systemic (vaginal) prostaglandin E_2
      a) Suppositories are inserted into vagina to induce abortion.
      b) Complications: nausea, vomiting, fever

5. Intrauterine (intra-amniotic) prostaglandin F_{2a}
   a) Prostaglandin F_{2a} is injected into amniotic sac to induce abortion.
   b) Complications: vomiting, fever, cervical rupture, bleeding, infection, delivery of live fetus
6. Hysterotomy
   a) Major surgery is done vaginally or abdominally after failure of abortion by other methods.
   b) Complications: morbidity, mortality, delivery of live fetus

C. Essential nursing care
   1. Nursing assessment
      a) Obtain history: medical, menstrual, contraceptive, obstetrical, previous abortion.
      b) Assist in physical examination to determine length of gestation, potential for complications, and medical conditions in which pregnancy causes danger to life of pregnant woman.
      c) Assist in diagnostic tests: pregnancy test, hemoglobin, hematocrit, Rh factor, STD screening, ultrasound.
      d) Assess client's knowledge of alternatives to abortion, of types of abortions, and of recovery process.
      e) Assess client's motivation for considering abortion.
      f) Assess client for presence of uncertainty, conflict, outside force, or distress.
   2. Nursing diagnoses
      a) Knowledge deficit related to:
         (1) Alternatives to abortion and to types of abortion procedures
         (2) Risks of abortion and to expected effects after abortion procedure
      b) Potential for infection related to procedure
      c) Pain related to procedure
      d) Ineffective individual coping related to anxiety or conflict about procedure
      e) Altered family processes related to stress caused by the decision
   3. Nursing intervention
      a) Present objective information about choices available: having abortion, keeping the baby, putting the baby up for adoption.
      b) Provide information about different abortion procedures and about risks associated with procedures.
      c) Provide emotional support.
      d) Assist client in resolving conflicts or confusion.
      e) Teach client about postprocedure effects.

4. Nursing evaluation
   a) Client understands pertinent information received about abortion procedures and alternatives to abortion.
   b) Client makes a decision and is comfortable with it.
   c) If client chooses abortion, the procedure succeeds and recovery is satisfactory.

IV. Contraception (family planning)

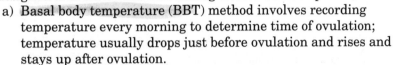

See text pages

A. Methods
   1. Natural family planning methods (fertility awareness methods designed to avoid intercourse during woman's fertile period)
      a) Basal body temperature (BBT) method involves recording temperature every morning to determine time of ovulation; temperature usually drops just before ovulation and rises and stays up after ovulation.
      b) Calendar (rhythm) method involves recording menstrual cycles over several months to determine fertile cycle and longest and shortest cycles in order to determine fertile period.
      c) Cervical mucus method involves daily assessment of changes in cervical mucus during menstrual cycle; cervical mucus present during fertile cycle is abundant, clear, and stretchable.
      d) Symptothermal method is a combination of the above fertility awareness methods.
      e) Advantages of natural family planning are that it is free; does not require artificial substances; does not interfere with most religious beliefs; is easily reversible; and has no side effects, complications, or contraindications.
      f) Disadvantages of natural family planning are that it interferes with spontaneity, requires periods of abstinence, may not be effective for client with irregular cycle, requires education to use properly, and requires much record keeping.
   2. Coitus interruptus (withdrawal)
      a) Advantages: is free; requires no artificial substances; has no side effects, complications, or contraindications
      b) Disadvantages: has a high failure rate and requires great self-control
   3. Hormonal contraception (pills or implants designed to inhibit ovulation by suppressing follicle stimulating hormone [FSH] or luteinizing hormone [LH])
      a) Types: combination pill (progestin and estrogen), minipill (progestin only), phasic oral contraceptives, morning-after pill (estrogen), subdermal implants (progestin)
      b) Advantages: highly effective, not related to intercourse, may give relief from menstrual pain

c) Disadvantages: does not protect against STDs and HIV infection, requires periodic visits to health care provider, can be expensive

d) Side effects: spotting, fluid retention, weight gain, breast tenderness, nausea, headaches, depression, excessive menstrual flow, breakthrough bleeding, clotting (see Client Teaching Checklist, "Danger Signs for Contraceptive Pill Use")

e) Complications: formation of blood clots, cardiovascular problems (stroke or heart attack), hypertension, cervical dysplasia

f) Contraindications: pregnancy; hypertension; diabetes; history of thrombophlebitis, thromboembolic disease, coronary artery disease, cancer of the breast or reproductive tract; heavy smoking; age over 40; migraine; liver disease; undiagnosed vaginal bleeding

4. Condom (sheaths of latex or lambskin placed over penis)
   a) Advantages: medically safe (no complications), inexpensive, available without prescription, effective in preventing STDs and decreasing the risk of AIDS (latex only)
   b) Disadvantages: highly subject to proper usage, related to intercourse, may break or become dislodged, decreased sensitivity to sexual feeling
   c) Side effects: allergic reaction and problems with erection
   d) Contraindications: allergy to latex or spermicide and cervical lesions

5. Vaginal sheath (female polyurethane condom)
   a) Advantages: safe (no known complications), available without prescription, may be inserted in advance of intercourse, may provide more protection against STDs than male condoms

---

✔ CLIENT TEACHING CHECKLIST ✔

Danger Signs for Contraceptive Pill Use

Clues for client:

✔ Abdominal pain (severe)
✔ Chest pains (severe) or shortness of breath
✔ Headaches (severe)
✔ Eye problems (blurred vision or loss of vision)
✔ Severe leg pain or swelling

b) Disadvantages: subject to proper usage and possible difficulty with insertion

c) Side effect: allergic reaction

d) Contraindications: allergy to latex or spermicide and cervical lesions

6. Vaginal spermicides

   a) Advantages: safe (no known complications) and simple to use

   b) Disadvantages: minimally effective when used alone; for some types, application 30 minutes before coitus during which client remains supine

   c) Side effect: allergy

   d) Contraindication: allergy

7. Diaphragm (rubber cap, used with spermicide, inserted into vagina before intercourse)

   a) Advantage: effective choice for client who cannot use contraceptive pill

   b) Disadvantages: requires fitting by health care provider, may have to be refitted after childbirth or weight gain or loss of more than 10 lb, interferes with spontaneity, requires proper insertion before intercourse to be effective

   c) Side effects: cramps, cystitis, allergic reaction, vaginitis

   d) Complications: possible occurrence of toxic shock syndrome (TSS), vaginal trauma

   e) Contraindications: history of TSS, abnormal vagina, urinary tract infection, severe pelvic pain

8. Cervical cap (rubber cap, used with spermicide, that fits over cervix)

   a) Advantage: effective choice for client who cannot use contraceptive pill

   b) Disadvantages: difficult to fit and more difficult to insert and remove than diaphragm

   c) Side effects: strong vaginal odor after 3 or 4 days and allergic reaction

   d) Complication: cervical trauma if too tight

   e) Contraindications: history of TSS, cervical infection, pelvic inflammatory disease (PID), cervicitis, abnormally shaped uterus or cervix, undiagnosed vaginal bleeding, abnormal Pap smear

9. Vaginal sponge (natural or synthetic sponge with spermicide)

   a) Advantages: no prescription or professional fitting needed, may be worn for up to 24 hours, may protect against STDs (chlamydial and gonorrheal infections)

   b) Disadvantages: difficult to remove and may cause irritation

   c) Side effect: allergic reaction

   d) Complication: possible occurrence of TSS

   e) Contraindications: history of TSS, vaginal abnormalities, allergy to materials

10. Intrauterine device (IUD) (mechanism inserted in uterine cavity to prevent pregnancy mainly by inducing an inflammatory response in the uterus)
    a) Advantages: continuous protection not related to intercourse and convenient, long-term effectiveness
    b) Disadvantages: requires fitting by health care provider, may be spontaneously expelled or dislodged, few on the market due to liability suits and to public's concern over complications, unacceptable to some clients because it may cause expulsion of zygote
    c) Side effects: pain during insertion, menstrual pain, increased menstrual bleeding, breakthrough bleeding, spotting (see Client Teaching Checklist, "Danger Signs for IUD Use")
    d) Complications: PID, perforation of uterus, syncope, ectopic pregnancy
    e) Contraindications: pelvic infection, pregnancy, impaired reaction to infection, heart valve disease, cervical cancer, multiple sex partners
11. Sterilization: permanent methods of contraception
    a) Vasectomy: surgical removal of part of vas deferens in male
        (1) Advantages: can be done on outpatient basis and has no effect on secondary sex characteristics
        (2) Disadvantages: difficult to reverse and results not immediate (Couple must use contraceptive until male reproductive tract is free of active sperm [about 6 weeks].)
        (3) Side effects: swelling and pain
        (4) Complications: hematoma, infection, discharge, painful granulomas
        (5) Contraindication: unsure about not wanting children

---

✔ CLIENT TEACHING CHECKLIST ✔

Danger Signs for IUD Use

Clues for client:

✔ Period (late or missed)
✔ Abdominal pain (severe)
✔ Increased temperature (fever) or chills
✔ Noticeable, foul-smelling discharge
✔ Spotting, bleeding, heavy periods, unusual clotting

b) Tubal ligation: surgical blocking of fallopian tubes in female
   (1) Advantage: can be done on outpatient basis
   (2) Disadvantage: difficult to reverse
   (3) Side effect: abdominal discomfort
   (4) Complications: bowel or uterine perforation, infection, hemorrhage, sterilization failure, reaction to anesthesia
   (5) Contraindication: unsure about not wanting children

B. Essential nursing care
   1. Nursing assessment
      a) Take history: menstrual, contraceptive, medical.
      b) Assess factors that influence choice of contraception: expense, preference, partner's support, frequency of intercourse, sexual practices, physical problems, religious or cultural factors.
      c) Assess client's knowledge of methods.
      d) Assess client for presence of contraindications for various types of contraception.
      e) Assess goals (motivation) for wanting to use contraception.
   2. Nursing diagnoses
      a) Knowledge deficit related to use of contraceptive method
      b) Potential for infection related to use of contraceptive method
      c) Potential for altered sexuality patterns related to loss of spontaneity
   3. Nursing intervention
      a) Explain methods: way to use, equipment required, advantages, requirements for method to be effective, effectiveness rates, side effects, possible complications.
      b) Clear up any misinformation client may have about methods.
      c) Provide client with information on proper way to use method of choice.
      d) Explain what to do if procedure for use is not followed.
      e) Provide client with information about what to do if a warning sign develops.
      f) Make sure informed consent is obtained prior to invasive procedure.
   4. Nursing evaluation
      a) Client understands how to use chosen method of contraception.
      b) Client is satisfied with chosen method of contraception.
      c) Client understands side effects and complications and knows warning signs.
      d) Client uses contraceptive method effectively and with no adverse reaction.
      e) Client demonstrates knowledge of what to do if warning signs develop.

1. Amelia Cruz is scheduled for an endometrial biopsy at the Fertility Clinic. The nurse understands that the best time for Mrs. Cruz to have the biopsy is during the:

   a. Follicular phase. *after ovulation*
   b. Luteal phase.
   c. Postcoital phase.
   d. Proliferative phase.

2. John and Alice Montrose are being seen at the Fertility Clinic. Which piece of data taken during the initial nursing assessment would be significant as a possible cause of infertility?

   a. Alice: onset of menses, age 12
   b. Alice: history of Pap Smear Class I
   c. John: history of appendectomy, age 28
   d. John: history of mumps, age 18

3. Clomiphene citrate (Clomid) is used primarily in the management of infertility to:

   a. Facilitate multiple births.
   b. Induce ovulation.
   c. Facilitate sperm motility.
   d. Increase sexual libido.

4. Maternal serum alpha-fetoprotein testing is done:

   a. Prior to pregnancy as a means of karyotyping.
   b. During the third trimester.
   c. As a screening tool for possible fetal abnormalities.
   d. As a predictor of fetal viability.

5. An amniocentesis has been ordered for Erin McKinley, age 41, primigravida, who is at 16 weeks' gestation. While preparing Mrs. McKinley for the amniocentesis, the nurse should:

   a. Obtain spouse's permission.
   b. Instruct Mrs. McKinley to empty her bladder prior to the test.
   c. Advise Mrs. McKinley about the need for bed rest for 24 hours following the test.
   d. Inform Mrs. McKinley that the results will be available within 48 hours.

6. Philip and Marisa Giotti are planning their first pregnancy. Marisa is very anxious and states, "My brother is a hemophiliac. Does that mean that my children will be hemophiliacs too?" The best response by the nurse is:

   a. "Mrs. Giotti, you may be a carrier. Let me explain how hemophilia is passed from mother to child."
   b. "Don't worry about it. Hemophilia is passed from father to son."
   c. "I can't answer that. Talk to your doctor about it."
   d. "You should know that all of your children will be carriers of the abnormal gene."

7. Sarah Melton, age 21, is about to be discharged from the Women's Health Center following an uncomplicated abortion. The nurse is evaluating Mrs. Melton's understanding of the discharge teaching. Which statement by Sarah indicates a need for further teaching?

   a. "I should report any temperature of 100.4°F or more to my caregiver."
   b. "I need to talk with my husband regarding no sexual intercourse for 2 weeks."
   c. "I'll miss not having a tub bath for the next 2 weeks."
   d. "I'll need to avoid exercise until my next period."

8. Rebecca Epstein, age 19, is at 16 weeks' gestation with her first pregnancy. While the nurse is completing the initial nursing assessment at an abortion clinic, Ms. Epstein says to the nurse, "I'm really ambivalent about abortion, but I don't know what else to do." The best nursing diagnosis for Ms. Epstein is:

   a. Self-concept disturbance related to abortion procedure.
   b. Altered family processes related to stress caused by decision to have abortion.

c. Potential for infection related to abortion procedure.

d. Knowledge deficit related to alternatives to abortion.

9. The nurse is discussing family-planning options with Molly Mendoza, age 38. Ms. Mendoza's history includes smoking, obesity, irregular menstrual cycles, and heavy menstrual flow. Which method would be safest yet most effective given Ms. Mendoza's history?

   a. Intrauterine device (IUD)
   b. Oral contraceptives
   c. Spermicides and condoms
   d. Natural family planning

10. Hypertension, thrombophlebitis, and breast cancer are contraindications for which of the following contraceptive methods?

    a. IUD
    b. Diaphragm
    c. Combination oral contraceptives
    d. Contraceptive sponge

11. Martha Williams, age 28, comes to the family-planning clinic requesting a diaphragm. Which piece of data obtained during the nursing interview would indicate to the nurse that Ms. Williams may not be a good candidate for a diaphragm?

    a. Client smokes a pack of cigarettes a day.
    b. Client has consistent sexual partner.
    c. Client has a history of urinary tract infection.
    d. Client is 6 weeks postpartum.

12. Frank Leedom is postop vasectomy. Discharge teaching for Mr. Leedom should include the following statement:

    a. For about 6 weeks, unprotected intercourse may lead to pregnancy.
    b. It is normal to experience hematuria for the first 24–48 hours.
    c. Often, secondary sex characteristics will decrease after a vasectomy.
    d. The vasectomy can be easily reversed during the first 6 weeks.

ANSWERS

1. **Correct answer is b.** An endometrial biopsy is done after ovulation has occurred. It identifies endometrial changes in response to ovulation.

   a. The follicular phase occurs in the ovarian cycle prior to ovulation.
   c. The postcoital phase is the time following intercourse.
   d. The proliferative phase occurs in the menstrual cycle prior to ovulation.

2. **Correct answer is d.** A history of mumps orchitis may be cause of male infertility.

   a and **b.** Both are normal findings in females.
   c. An appendectomy should not cause infertility.

3. **Correct answer is b.** Clomid stimulates the release of pituitary gonadotropins FSH and LH, resulting in ovulation and the development of the corpus luteum.

   a. Although a side effect of Clomid is multiple births, that is not the primary use in infertility.
   c. Clomid does not facilitate sperm motility directly. Changes in cervical mucus do occur with ovulation, which may or may not facilitate sperm motility.
   d. Clomid has no direct effect on increasing sexual drive.

4. **Correct answer is c.** Alpha-fetoprotein testing is primarily a screening test for possible fetal neural tube defects.

   a. Alpha-fetoprotein testing is not a prepregnancy test.
   b. Alpha-fetoprotein testing is not done during the third trimester. It is usually completed during 15–18 weeks of gestation.
   d. Alpha-fetoprotein testing is not done to determine fetal viability.

5. **Correct answer is b.** Bladder is emptied to prevent bladder puncture.

   a. The spouse's permission is not required.
   c. There is no need for 24-hour bed rest. Mrs. McKinley would be asked to rest for 1–2 hours.
   d. Results take 7 days to 4 weeks.

6. **Correct answer is a.** Mrs. Giotti may indeed be a carrier. Mrs. Giotti's mother is the carrier for the abnormal gene received by Mrs. Giotti's brother. Statistically, one-half of all the daughters of a carrier mother will be carriers.

   b. Hemophilia is an X-linked recessive trait (the abnormal gene is carried on the X chromosome). Hemophiliac males cannot pass the abnormal gene to sons, only to daughters.
   c. This response does not answer Mrs. Giotti's questions and would only add to her anxiety. Nurses are well prepared to discuss such topics.
   d. If Mrs. Giotti is a carrier, there is a *50%* chance of each of her *female* children being a carrier.

7. **Correct answer is d.** There is no need to eliminate moderate exercise or Mrs. Melton's usual exercise program. If she begins to have increased blood flow, she will have to contact her caregiver.

   a, b, and **c.** All are correct statements by Mrs. Melton, indicating an understanding of her discharge teaching.

8. **Correct answer is d.** Ms. Epstein's statement indicates a lack of understanding of alternatives available for her.

   a. There are no data to support difficulty with self-concept.
   b. She has not yet made a decision for abortion.
   c. Potential for infection would be a consideration only if she does have an abortion.

9. **Correct answer is c.** Given Ms. Mendoza's history, use of spermicides and condoms is the only choice for which there are no contraindications.

   a. A history of heavy menstrual flow would prohibit the IUD.
   b. Smoking is contraindicated with oral contraceptives. Also, her age may be a factor.
   d. Irregular menstrual cycles may make natural family planning difficult and ineffective.

10. **Correct answer is c.** Oral contraceptives containing estrogen are contraindicated for women with high blood pressure, a history of thrombophlebitis, or known or suspected breast cancer.

    a, b, and **d.** Hypertension, thrombophlebitis, and breast cancer are not contraindications for IUD, diaphragm, or sponge.

11. **Correct answer is c.** Increased pressure from a diaphragm on the urethra may interfere with complete bladder emptying and lead to recurrent urinary tract infections.

    a. Smoking does not relate to the use of a diaphragm.
    b and **d.** These issues do not present a problem for use of a diaphragm.

12. **Correct answer is a.** Following a vasectomy, it will take 4–6 weeks to clear remaining active sperm from vas deferens.

    b. Mr. Leedom should not experience bloody urine. If he does, he should notify his physician.
    c. Secondary sex characteristics will not decrease as a result of vasectomy.
    d. Vasectomy is not easily reversed.

5

Normal Pregnancy

1. Virtually all body systems are affected by pregnancy and return almost completely to normal after delivery and lactation.
2. Metabolism and distribution of nutrients tend to favor needs of the fetus.
3. Women experience predictable and sequential phases in adapting to pregnancy; other family members go through similar adjustments.
4. Nurse can provide reassurance during client's pregnancy through counseling, teaching, and emotional support.
5. Anticipatory guidance from nurse can help identify discomforts of pregnancy and provide methods to ease or alleviate them.
6. Nurse should be aware throughout the client's pregnancy of danger signals.
7. Most clients require dietary modification to meet the needs of pregnancy.
8. Fetus is affected by mother's nutritional status.
9. Nurse should consider impact of factors such as age, parity, food preferences, financial status, and culture on the client's dietary selections.
10. Nurse should take into account and respect the learning needs of clients with respect to childbirth education.

GLOSSARY

ballottement—technique of detecting passive movements of unengaged fetus as it floats in amniotic fluid

Braxton Hicks contractions—irregular, mild uterine contractions that occur throughout pregnancy; may be confused with true labor late in pregnancy

effleurage—massage of abdomen with fingertips

funic souffle—sound of fetal blood coursing through umbilical cord

gravida—pregnant woman

Kegel exercises—exercises to strengthen pubococcygeal muscles through tightening and relaxing

multigravida—woman who has been pregnant more than once

multipara—woman who has given birth to more than 1 viable infant

myometrium—muscular layer of uterine wall

nulligravida—woman who has never been pregnant

nullipara—woman who has not given birth to a viable infant (para 0)

primigravida—woman pregnant for the first time (gravida 1)

primipara—woman who has given birth to 1 viable infant (para 1)

quickening—perception by mother of fetal movement

uterine souffle—soft blowing or whizzing sound heard over uterus; caused by blood rushing through large vessels to placenta, synchronous with maternal pulse

I. Biophysical changes

A. Uterus

1. First trimester
   a) Uterine isthmus softens (Hegar's sign).
   b) Myometrial cells increase in size (hypertrophy).
   c) New muscle fibers and fibroelastic tissue are produced (hyperplasia).
2. Second trimester
   a) Uterus rises out of pelvis and is palpable at symphysis pubis. (third–fourth month)
   b) Uterus reaches umbilicus. (sixth month)
   c) Shape of uterus changes from spherical to globular.
   d) Blood vessels and lymphatic channels become dilated and increasingly vascular, causing pelvic congestion and edema.
   e) Uterine walls become thicker, stronger, and elastic.
3. Third trimester
   a) Shape changes to ovoid as uterus rises out of pelvis into abdominal cavity.
   b) Uterus impinges on xiphoid process. (ninth month)

B. Cervix

1. Tip of the cervix softens (Goodell's sign) and feels like an earlobe.
2. Mucus plug (operculum) seals endocervical canal from contamination by vaginal bacteria.
3. Cervix takes on a blue-purple discoloration (Chadwick's sign). (sixth week)

C. Ovaries

1. Ovaries become quiescent as follicular activity is suppressed.
2. Corpus luteum continues to produce estrogen and progesterone until placental production occurs. (8–10 weeks)

D. Vagina

1. The mucosa thickens, and connective tissue loosens.
2. Secretions increase, and their pH becomes acidic to prevent infection.
3. Vagina becomes increasingly sensitive, often leading to a woman's increased sexual interest and arousal.
4. Vagina relaxes at the end of pregnancy to permit passage of fetus.

E. Breasts

1. Breasts increase in both size and nodularity because of glandular hyperplasia and hypertrophy that occur in preparation for lactation.
2. Breasts become tender, heavy, and full, with heightened sensitivity and tingling.
3. Nipples and areolae become more pigmented, with the appearance of secondary pinkish areolae.

See text pages
_____

       4. Sebaceous glands embedded in the areolae become enlarged (Montgomery's tubercles).

       5. Superficial veins become more prominent.

       6. Thin, clear, viscous secretion (colostrum) can be expressed from nipples. (as early as 12–14 weeks)

         a) Contains the immunoglobulin secretory IgA

         b) Will provide neonate's immunological defense against gastrointestinal bacteria

   F. Cardiovascular system

       1. Heart becomes hypertrophied and pushed upward, to the left, and rotated forward from fetal pressure on diaphragm.

       2. Blood flow is increased to kidneys, uterus, and skin.

       3. Pulse rate increases; palpitations may occur.

       4. Blood volume increases by about 40%, with increased production of red blood cells to transport additional oxygen.

         a) Hemoglobin and hematocrit values decrease.

         b) Physiologic anemia of pregnancy (pseudoanemia) develops due to disproportionate increase in blood volume compared with number of red blood cells.

         c) Iron levels may be insufficient because of increased demand during production of red blood cells (can be treated with dietary supplementation).

         d) White cells increase (leukocytosis).

       5. Increased fibrin and fibrinogen levels lead to decreased ability to dissolve clots.

         a) Results in hypercoagulable state of pregnancy

         b) Increased risk of client's developing venous thrombosis

         c) Exacerbated by venous stasis or decreased venous return from lower extremities

       6. Blood pressure decreases to lowest point in second trimester because of increased cardiac output and reduced peripheral resistance; returns to normal in third trimester.

         a) Femoral venous pressure rises as gravid uterus exerts pressure on return of blood flow.

           (1) Venous congestion leads to varicose veins and hemorrhoids.

           (2) Client may develop postural hypotension.

         b) Blood pressure falls when client is in supine position, causing vena caval, or supine hypotensive, syndrome.

           (1) Enlarged uterus presses on vena cava, obstructing return blood flow.

           (2) Fetal heart rate slows.

           (3) Client becomes dizzy, pale, and clammy.

           (4) Hypotension can be corrected by client lying on her left side.

G. Respiratory system
   1. Tidal volume (air breathed with each respiration) increases as client breathes deeper.
      a) Results in hyperventilation of pregnancy
      b) Influenced by progesterone, which makes the respiratory center more sensitive to carbon dioxide
   2. Respiratory rate (breaths per minute) does not change.
   3. Total body oxygen consumption increases (15%–20%) to meet increased maternal and fetal demands.
   4. Decreased airway resistance increases oxygen consumption.
   5. Dyspnea occurs in third trimester due to uterine enlargement.
   6. Diaphragm is elevated, with rib cage flaring.
   7. Vascular congestion and edema increase in upper respiratory tract.
      a) Influenced by circulating estrogen
      b) Results in nasal and sinus stuffiness and nosebleeds

H. Gastrointestinal system
   1. Blood vessels in gums become swollen (epulis of pregnancy).
   2. Salivation increases and may become excessive (ptyalism).
   3. Stomach is displaced upward.
      a) Hiatal hernia can occur.
      b) Heartburn (pyrosis) results from reflux of stomach acid into lower esophagus through relaxed cardiac sphincter in diaphragm.
   4. Constipation occurs.
      a) Affected by delayed gastric emptying time, decreased gastric motility, decrease in tone of intestinal muscles, increased water reabsorption in colon, atypical food selection, increased appetite and, possibly, by iron supplementation
      b) Predisposes to formation of hemorrhoids
   5. Liver changes occur: Small alterations in laboratory tests for hepatic function occur; they would be abnormal for nonpregnant woman but are normal for pregnant woman.
   6. Gallbladder changes occur.
      a) Tone decreases; distention increases.
      b) Hypercholesterolemia occurs from the influence of progesterone, possibly resulting in gallstones of pregnancy.
   7. Cumulative intra-abdominal alterations cause flatulence, cramping, and bloating.

I. Urinary tract
   1. Enlarging uterus places pressure on bladder, causing urinary frequency until uterus grows out of pelvis.
   2. Ureters (right more than left) become dilated, especially at pelvic brim.
      a) Larger volume of urine is held in renal pelvises and ureters.
      b) Urinary stasis develops, causing increased susceptibility to urinary tract infection.

3. Bladder sensitivity and compression increases, causing nocturia, urinary frequency, and urinary urgency (without dysuria) in early pregnancy.
4. Renal function is altered significantly.
   a) Glomerular filtration rate (GFR) and renal plasma flow (RPF) increase.
   b) Plasma creatinine and blood urea nitrogen (BUN) levels decrease.
   c) Selective renal tubular reabsorption of sodium and water increases.
   d) Impaired tubular reabsorption of glucose occurs, leading to glycosuria.
      (1) Increased sugar levels in urine may not be pathogenic.
      (2) Possibility of presence of diabetes must be investigated through serum testing.
   e) Trace protein in urine may occur, but measurable amount of protein is a sign of renal disease or toxemia.

J. Integumentary system
   1. Changes in pigmentation: caused by increase in hormone melanotropin
      a) Linea nigra: black line from symphysis pubis to top of fundus along the body's midline
      b) Chloasma (mask of pregnancy): brown blotches or irregular facial spots, which are accentuated by sun exposure
   2. Striae gravidarum (stretch marks)
      a) Separation of underlying connective tissue due to elevated levels of adrenal steroids
      b) Appear on abdomen, thighs, and breasts
   3. Spider hemangiomas
      a) Minute red blemishes with branching legs
      b) Caused by elevated levels of circulating estrogen
      c) May be accompanied by palmar erythema (diffuse redness on palms)
   4. Thinning and softening of fingernails and toenails
   5. Oily skin and acne vulgaris caused by increased activity of sebaceous and sweat glands
   6. Hair growth
      a) Growth of fine hair increases (hirsutism).
      b) Hair may also be thicker and more abundant.

K. Musculoskeletal system
   1. Posture changes from increased anterior uterine weight.
      a) Client's center of gravity shifts.
      b) Abdominal distention gives pelvis forward tilt.

     c) Lumbosacral spinal curve becomes accentuated.

     d) Changes frequently cause low back pain.

  2. Sacroiliac, sacrococcygeal, and pubic joints relax and become increasingly mobile.

     a) Causes waddling gait of pregnancy

     b) Permits enlargement of pelvic dimensions

  3. Abdominal muscles stretch and lose tone.

     a) Rectus abdominis muscles may separate (diastasis recti).

     b) Umbilicus protrudes or flattens.

L. Endocrine system

  1. Placental hormones (see Chapter 3, section VI,A,6, for functions of hormones secreted by placenta)

  2. Thyroid gland

     a) Enlargement of gland is caused by cellular hyperplasia and increased vascularity but is not associated with increased thyroid activity.

     b) Basal metabolic rate (BMR) increases, caused by increased oxygen consumption for fetal metabolic activity.

  3. Parathyroid gland

     a) Slight secondary hyperparathyroidism occurs, peaking between 15 and 35 weeks.

     b) Increased activity parallels fetal calcium requirements.

  4. Pituitary gland

     a) Anterior lobe

        (1) Secretion of gonadotropins (follicle stimulating hormone [FSH] and luteinizing hormone [LH]) is inhibited by placental production of estrogen and progesterone during pregnancy.

        (2) Production of thyrotropin and adrenotropin is increased: responsible for altering maternal metabolism to support pregnancy.

        (3) Production of prolactin is responsible for initiating lactation.

     b) Posterior lobe

        (1) Production of oxytocin promotes uterine contractility and stimulates milk ejection from breasts. Oxytocin levels increase as gestation progresses to term.

        (2) Production of vasopressin causes vasoconstriction (increases blood pressure) and antidiuresis.

  5. Adrenal glands

     a) Circulating cortisol levels increase, regulating carbohydrate and protein metabolism.

     b) Production of aldosterone helps regulate blood sodium levels and helps increase blood volume through retention of sodium and water.

  6. Pancreas

     a) Increased cortisol, gonadotropins, and human placental lactogen (hPL) decrease client's ability to use insulin.

     b) Maternal insulin resistance ensures ample supply of glucose for fetus.

        c) Pancreatic islets of Langerhans are stressed to increase insulin production.

        d) Preexisting marginal pancreatic function may become gestational diabetes.

M. Metabolic changes

1. Weight gain (24–30 lb recommended): most associated with products of conception (fetus, placenta, amniotic fluid)
2. Water retention: results from increase in hormones responsible for sodium and fluid retention and lowered serum protein
3. Modification of metabolism of nutrients to meet fetal demands (greatest during second half of pregnancy)
   a) Increased retention of nitrogen (protein)
   b) Increased absorption of fats, leading to increased serum levels of lipids, lipoproteins, and cholesterol
   c) Increased demand for carbohydrates and iron
   d) Absorption and retention of calcium

II. Psychologic changes to client and family

A. Maternal adaptation

1. First trimester
   a) Ambivalence
   b) Fear
   c) Fantasies about motherhood and about having a "dream" child
   d) Possible decrease in sex drive due to physical discomforts (nausea and fatigue)
2. Second trimester
   a) Alternate feelings of emotional well-being and lability (rapid mood swings)
   b) Acceptance of pregnancy as coinciding with decrease in nausea and fatigue and with onset of quickening
   c) Possible increase in sex drive, associated with physical well-being
   d) Adjustment to change in body image as gradual loss of body boundaries occurs
   e) Possible occurrence of introversion and introspection
3. Third trimester
   a) Feelings of awkwardness and clumsiness
   b) Renewed fears and tensions about labor and wellness of fetus
   c) Increased nesting behavior
   d) Spurt of energy during last month
4. Tasks of pregnant woman
   a) Incorporating fetus into her own bodily image

See text pages

b) Accepting adult responsibilities: rite of passage signifying reaching maturity
c) Identifying with motherhood role
d) Perceiving fetus as separate object
e) Developing bonds of love
f) Readying herself to assume caretaking relationship
g) Preparing for physical separation (birth of the infant)

B. Paternal adaptation
1. Phases of adaptation
a) Announcement phase: accepts biologic fact of pregnancy but may begin to feel left out
b) Moratorium phase: adjusts to the reality of the pregnancy
(1) His involvement is facilitated by feeling fetal movement.
(2) He responds to woman's physical changes and may have alteration of sexual interest.
c) Focusing phase: evolution of more clearly defined role (e.g., concern with how to participate in labor and prepare for parenthood)
2. Paternal readiness for pregnancy: related to sense of financial security, stability in the couple's relationship, and closure of childless period in relationship

C. Adaptation of family members
1. Siblings: experience rivalry because of fear of change in relationship with parents
2. Grandparents: are often unsure about level of involvement

III. Methods of determining pregnancy

See text pages
_____

A. Presumptive signs of pregnancy: menstrual suppression, nausea and vomiting, frequent urination, breast changes, excessive fatigue, quickening

B. Probable (objective) signs of pregnancy
1. Abdominal enlargement
2. Uterine softening and enlargement
a) Softening of lower part of uterus (Hegar's sign): 6–8 weeks
b) General growth and softening: after 8 weeks
3. Ballottement
4. Softening of the cervix (Goodell's sign) and discoloration of the cervix (Chadwick's sign)
5. Presence of Braxton Hicks contractions beginning early in pregnancy
6. Souffle

C. Positive (diagnostic) signs of pregnancy: 100% accurate
1. Fetal heartbeat: detected with a fetoscope by approximately 17–20 weeks; can detect at 10–12 weeks with Doppler device; normal between 120 and 160 beats per minute
2. Fetal movement: palpable by trained examiner at 20 weeks

3. Fetus detected by ultrasound: useful as early as sixth week; especially useful at 16–18 weeks to date pregnancy precisely

D. Pregnancy tests: involve measurement of early human chorionic gonadotropin (hCG) secreted by the chorionic villi of implanted ovum; may be a probable or positive sign of pregnancy, depending on test
   1. Immunoassay tests: detect hCG in maternal blood or urine
      a) Agglutination-inhibition test: no clumping of cells occurs when maternal urine is added to hCG-sensitized red blood cells of sheep; 95% accurate; detects pregnancy 10–14 days after first missed menses
      b) Latex agglutination tests: latex particle agglutination is inhibited in the presence of maternal urine with hCG; 95% accurate; detect pregnancy 10–14 days after first missed menses
      c) Radioimmunoassay (RIA): blood test that detects pregnancy a few days after conception; uses antiserum with specificity for the beta subunit antibody of hCG in blood plasma
      d) Enzyme immunoassay: detects beta hCG in urine or serum; takes a few minutes to perform; can detect pregnancy before first missed period; not subject to cross-reactions
   2. Radioreceptor assay (RRA): identifies hCG in maternal blood; accurate within 14 days of conception; also registers positive when it identifies LH; requires sophisticated equipment
   3. Home pregnancy tests: performed on urine; use beta subunit antibody or agglutination-inhibition principle; have high false-negative rate in very early pregnancy (up to 25% if performed less than 14 days after conception)

See text pages

IV. Essential antepartal nursing care during initial prenatal visit

A. Determining due date: also known as estimated date of delivery (EDD) or estimated date of birth (EDB)
   1. Nägele's rule: add 7 days to the first date of the last menstrual period (LMP), subtract 3 months, add 1 year
   2. McDonald's rule: measurement of fundal height
      a) Height of fundus (cm) × 2/7 = gestation in lunar months
      b) Height of fundus (cm) × 8/7 = gestation in weeks
   3. Ultrasonography determinations
      a) Dimensions of gestational sac (as early as 6–10 weeks)
      b) Crown-to-rump length (7–14 weeks)
      c) Femur length (12 weeks)
      d) Biparietal diameter of fetal head (after 12 weeks)

B. Assessment (The role of the nurse in the assessment phase is determined by level of training, experience, and care setting.)
   1. Maternal history
      a) Current pregnancy: Identify first day of LMP and any discomfort since LMP; identify client's attitude toward pregnancy and her opinion about when conception occurred.
      b) Past pregnancies: Identify number of prior pregnancies, abortions, and living children; history of prior pregnancies including labor and delivery; perinatal status of previous children; maternal blood type and Rh factor; and previous prenatal education.
      c) Gynecologic history: Identify past infections, surgeries, menstrual history, sexual history, method of contraception, date of last Pap smear, and history of any Pap smear abnormalities.
      d) Current medical history: Identify status of general health, medications taken, habits (smoking, alcohol, illicit drug use/abuse), allergies, teratogenic exposure, current health problems, and immunization history (especially rubella).
      e) Past medical history: Identify childhood diseases, surgery, past illnesses, hospitalizations, bleeding disorders, and history of blood transfusion; perform review of systems.
      f) Family medical history: Identify health status of parents and siblings, history of illnesses (diabetes, hypertension, cardiovascular or hematologic disorders), prior multiple births, and congenital deformities.
      g) Personal history: Identify religion/cultural background, occupation, living conditions, economic status, support system, attitudes and information about childbirth, and emotional disturbances.
      h) Partner's history: Identify genetic conditions/diseases, age, health, alcohol or drug use, smoking, occupation, and attitude toward pregnancy.
   2. Relevant laboratory tests
      a) Urine
         (1) Analysis: to determine abnormal levels of sugar (glycosuria), a screen for diabetes; to determine abnormal levels of albumin (proteinuria), a screen for preeclampsia or renal problems
         (2) Microscopic examination: to evaluate red and white blood cells, epithelial cells, and casts as a screen for renal disease; to evaluate microorganisms as a screen for infection
         (3) Culture: to diagnose urinary tract infections
      b) Blood
         (1) Hemoglobin/hematocrit: to screen for anemia
         (2) White blood cell count, differential: to screen for infection and hematologic abnormalities
         (3) Blood type, Rh factor: to identify fetus at risk for Rh incompatibility (erythroblastosis fetalis)

      (4) Rh titer: to determine baseline values of Rh-negative mother and Rh-positive father (rising titers in mother signify danger to fetus)

      (5) Rubella titer: to determine immunity to rubella

      (6) Serologic tests for syphilis (VDRL, RPR, STS)

      (7) FTA-ABS (fluorescent treponemal antibody absorption test): to identify client with untreated syphilis

      (8) HIV antibody assay and hepatitis B antigen: to determine evidence of infection with HIV or hepatitis B

      (9) Glucose: to screen for gestational diabetes

    (10) Blood urea nitrogen (BUN), creatinine, total protein, electrolytes: to evaluate renal function

    (11) Hemoglobin electrophoresis: to screen for hemoglobinopathies (sickle cell anemia and thalassemias)

   c) Cervix/vagina

      (1) Culture of cervical discharge: to diagnose gonorrhea and *Chlamydia trachomatis*

      (2) Pap smear: to screen for cervical intraepithelial neoplasia, herpes simplex type 2, and human papillomaviruses

   d) Tuberculin skin testing: to screen high-risk clients for tuberculosis

  3. Physical examination

   a) Vital signs: Blood pressure, pulse, respiration, and temperature are taken.

   b) Weight: Baseline is established; rapid, sudden weight gain is noted; need for nutritional counseling is evaluated.

   c) Skin: Color, condition, lesions, and pigmentation are noted.

   d) Head and neck: Character and color of mucosa and presence of lymphadenopathy or thyroid enlargement or tenderness are noted.

   e) Chest and heart: Lung sounds and heart rhythms are noted.

   f) Breasts: Size and vascular patterns are inspected; masses, nodules, nipple discharge, lesions, and erythema are noted.

   g) Extremities: Ankle or pretibial edema, limitations of motion, varicosities, and reflexes are noted.

   h) Abdomen: Uterine size, presence of contractions, and enlarged liver or spleen are noted.

   i) Spine: Deformities, posture, and tenderness are noted.

   j) Pelvis

      (1) External inspection: Inspection is made for sexual maturity, clitoris, and labia; scars, inflammation, or lesions in the perineum are noted; presence of hemorrhoids is noted.

(2) External palpation: Inspection is made of urethra and Skene's and Bartholin's glands; discharges are cultured; vaginal orifice is examined; support of anterior and posterior vaginal walls is assessed.

(3) Internal inspection of cervix with speculum: Position, color, appearance of os, lesions, bleeding, and discharge are noted; as speculum is withdrawn, vaginal walls are observed for color, lesions, rugae (folds), fistulas, and bulging.

(4) Collection of specimens

    (a) Pap smear: Cervical spatula is placed in cervical os and rotated 360° to adequately sample surface of squamocolumnar junction; specimen is spread on slide, sprayed with fixative, and dried.

    (b) Gonorrhea culture: Specimen is obtained from endocervical canal using sterile applicator, rolled on culture plate (with special Thayer-Martin medium), and incubated.

    (c) *Chlamydia trachomatis* smear: Smears are obtained if urethral or cervical discharge is present; slides are incubated with fluorescein-labeled antibodies for 30 minutes, then examined.

    (d) Herpes simplex, types 1 and 2 culture: Culture is obtained from open lesion.

(5) Bimanual examination

    (a) Pointer finger and middle finger of one hand are lubricated and inserted into vagina to palpate for distensibility, lesions, and tenderness.

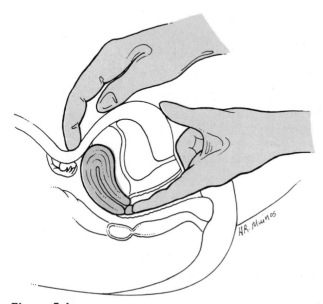

Figure 5-1
Bimanual Examination of Uterus

        (b) Cervix is examined for position, shape, consistency, mobility, and lesions.

        (c) The other hand is placed on abdomen between umbilicus and symphysis pubis; pressure is exerted down toward hand in pelvis, allowing reproductive structures to be assessed.

        (d) Uterus is assessed for position, size, shape, consistency, regularity, motility, masses, and tenderness.

        (e) With one hand on right lower quadrant of abdomen and other hand placed in pelvis on right lateral fornix, adnexa is assessed for position, size, tenderness, and masses; assessment is repeated on left side.

        (f) Pelvic measurements are taken.

      (6) Rectovaginal palpation

        (a) Index finger is inserted into vagina and middle finger into rectum.

        (b) Maneuvers of bimanual exam are repeated.

        (c) Rectovaginal septum, posterior surface of the uterus, and region behind the cervix are assessed.

    4. Identification of risk factors (see Chapter 6, sections I, II, and III, for discussion of risk factors in pregnancy)

  C. Nursing diagnoses

    1. Knowledge deficit related to:

      a) Emotional and physiologic changes of pregnancy

      b) Course of prenatal care

      c) Self-care during pregnancy

      d) Family adaptations to pregnancy

      e) Tests and procedures

      f) Signs and symptoms, potential danger to mother and fetus

    2. Altered nutrition, less than body requirements, related to nausea and vomiting (see section VI,E of this chapter for other nutritional diagnoses)

    3. Potential for anxiety related to:

      a) Client's concern about herself and her safety

      b) Physical changes of pregnancy

      c) Emotional aspects of pregnancy

    4. Altered comfort related to early discomforts of pregnancy

    5. Altered family processes related to:

      a) Family's response to diagnosis of pregnancy

      b) Need for different coping strategies

      c) Need for role adjustments

6. Altered sexuality patterns related to:
   a) Early discomforts of pregnancy
   b) Emotional reactions to pregnancy
   c) Fear of harming the baby
7. Ineffective family coping related to:
   a) Emotional disturbances
   b) Inadequate financial resources

D. Nursing intervention
1. Interview client and gain information for the prenatal health assessment; explain normal physiologic and psychologic adaptations to pregnancy.
2. Provide overview of the process of prenatal care; inform client of schedule for prenatal visits: once a month until the seventh month, every 2 weeks during the seventh and eighth months, and weekly during the ninth month until delivery.
3. Discuss current problems and provide education for self-care related to:
   a) Nausea and vomiting
      (1) Avoid the odor of certain foods or other conditions that precipitate the problem.
      (2) Eat crackers or dry toast before arising slowly.
      (3) Avoid sudden position changes.
      (4) Eat small, frequent meals.
      (5) Avoid greasy or highly seasoned foods.
      (6) Avoid antiemetics during first trimester because of danger of teratogenic effects.
   b) Nasal stuffiness and epistaxis
      (1) Use cool-air vaporizers and normal saline drops.
      (2) Avoid nasal sprays and decongestants (possible addiction and eventual rebound effect).
   c) Breast tenderness: Wear well-fitting supportive bra.
   d) Increased vaginal discharge
      (1) Bathe daily.
      (2) Avoid douching and nylon underwear.
      (3) Wear pantyhose with cotton crotch.
   e) Ptyalism: Use astringent mouthwashes, chew gum, or suck hard candy.
   f) Urinary frequency
      (1) Void when urge is felt.
      (2) Increase fluid intake during the day and decrease fluid intake only in the evening.
4. Explain different roles and adaptations family members may make in response to the pregnancy.
5. Explain the reasons for the different tests, how they are done, and what to expect.

6. Describe danger signs of complications to the client: vaginal bleeding, abdominal cramping, persistent and frequent nausea and vomiting, chills, fever, swelling of face or fingers, dimmed or blurred vision, and severe headaches.

7. Stress to the client that successful completion of the pregnancy is related to a combination of good physical and emotional health as well as avoidance of activities or behaviors that may be detrimental to the fetus.

8. Identify practices that promote maternal and fetal well-being and prevent complications:
   a) Prevention of urinary tract infections: includes adequate cleansing, increased fluid intake, and frequent bladder emptying
   b) Exercise
      (1) Regular schedule of walking
      (2) Sports: must be considered carefully because of changes in client's gait, balance, and center of gravity
      (3) Specific prenatal exercises
         (a) Abdominal muscle tightening in synchronization with respiration
         (b) Kegel's perineal exercises for strengthening the pelvic floor (see Client Teaching Checklist, "Kegel Exercises")
         (c) Pelvic tilt exercises to alleviate backache and to strengthen abdominal muscles
   c) Avoidance of cigarettes, alcohol, and drugs
   d) Avoidance of immunizations unless recommended by health care provider

9. Teach the client about the importance of nutrition and modifications to make if nausea and vomiting occur.

10. Reassure the client that her concerns are normal and that she will be given information to help allay her fears.

11. Instruct client about measures to relieve early discomfort:
    a) Improve posture to relieve lower or upper backache.
    b) Allow for increased time for sleep or naps.
    c) Minimize ankle edema by resting with feet elevated.
    d) Participate in appropriate level of physical activity.

12. Describe the different responses family members have to the pregnancy and stress that coping strategies and role adjustments may be necessary.

13. Counsel the client about sexual activity during pregnancy.
    a) Couples should be reassured that their concerns are normal.
    b) Sexual activity need not be limited unless there is bleeding or ruptured membranes.
    c) Sexual desires may change throughout pregnancy.
    d) Sexual intimacy needs to include practices other than intercourse.

Kegel Exercises

Explanation of 3 types of Kegel exercises to client:

1. Alternately squeeze and relax pubococcygeal muscle (muscle that is tensed to stop urinary flow while voiding) for 3 seconds at a time.
   - ✔ Begin with a series of 10 squeezes once a day.
   - ✔ Increase until doing a series of 10 several times a day.
2. Squeeze and release pubococcygeal muscle rapidly and repeatedly.
3. Pull up pelvic floor, then bear down as if doing a bowel movement but using vaginal muscles instead of rectal muscles.

Purposes of exercises:

- ✔ To improve urine retention
- ✔ To increase elasticity and contractility of perineal and vaginal muscles
- ✔ To improve support to pelvic organs

Special notes:

- ✔ Exercises are most effective when muscles of buttocks and thighs are not used.
- ✔ Exercises should not be done while urinating—may cause infection.
- ✔ Exercises can be done anytime and anywhere (e.g., sitting in a car, standing on line, reading).

14. Provide ways in which families may work together to resolve emotional conflicts.
15. Help the family investigate opportunities for increasing financial resources or more effectively using current funds.

E. Nursing evaluation
   1. Client understands the normal psychologic and physiologic variations of pregnancy.
   2. Client is aware of the prenatal evaluation process and the schedule of visits that will be necessary.
   3. Client understands self-care methods.
   4. Client is informed that family members may respond differently to the pregnancy, which may require adaptations and role changes.
   5. Client understands the tests and why they are necessary.
   6. Client is able to identify the signs that may indicate danger to herself or the fetus.
   7. Client appreciates that regular prenatal care and good health practices will enhance the chance for the delivery of a healthy baby.
   8. Client is reassured about the safety of the fetus and what she can emotionally and physically expect.
   9. Client knows how to treat discomfort she may feel.
   10. Client is reassured and knowledgeable about sexual activity.
   11. Family is able to secure additional income or use current resources more efficiently.

See text pages

_____

V. Essential nursing care during follow-up prenatal visits

A. Assessment
  1. Maternal assessment
     a) Interview: Client is asked for summary of events since last visit (general well-being and complaints or problems) and for any questions she may have.
     b) Physical examination
        (1) Vital signs, with special attention given to blood pressure
           (a) Significant: systolic blood pressure ≥140 mm Hg; diastolic blood pressure ≥90 mm Hg
           (b) Significant, regardless of whether absolute values are less than 140/90: rise in systolic pressure of ≥30 over baseline and rise in diastolic pressure of ≥15
        (2) Weight: Determine whether weight gain or loss is compatible with overall plan for weight gain.
  2. Fetal assessment
     a) Fundal height: used to assess fetal growth; may help identify high-risk conditions
     b) Fetal movement: Woman is asked to note time and duration of fetal movements (see Client Teaching Checklist, "Methods of Assessment of Fetal Activity by Pregnant Woman").
     c) Fetal heart rate: done with stethoscope, fetoscope, or Doppler device
  3. Laboratory and diagnostic tests
     a) Urinalysis is done each visit.
     b) Other routine tests from initial visit are repeated only as indicated.
     (See Chapter 6, section IV, for description of tests used in high-risk pregnancies [e.g., chorionic villus sampling and amniocentesis].)

B. Nursing diagnoses
  1. Knowledge deficit related to:
     a) Self-care to reduce discomfort
     b) Preparation for labor and delivery
     c) Danger signals
  2. Potential for anxiety related to:
     a) Discomforts of pregnancy
     b) Fetal well-being
  3. Potential for injury related to nonuse of safety belt in automobiles

C. Nursing intervention
  1. Instruct client in ways to treat problems and provide comfort.
     a) Heartburn (pyrosis): Limit gas-producing or fatty foods and maintain good posture.

Methods of Assessment of Fetal Activity by Pregnant Woman

Explanation to client:

✔ Starting at end of sixth month, monitor fetal movement daily.
  — For normal pregnancy: Count fetal movements 2 times each day for a period of 20–30 minutes each time; 5 or 6 movements are desirable in each counting period.
  — For high-risk pregnancy: Count fetal movements 3 times a day for 30 minutes each time; 5 or 6 movements are desirable. If count is low, count for 1 hour while lying down (3 or more movements are desirable in this count).
✔ Best times to count are 1 hour after eating and while resting, lying on side.
✔ Make a record of movements on a chart.

Causes for concern:

✔ Fewer than 10 movements in a 12-hour period (particularly during daytime hours)
✔ No movements in the morning
✔ Fewer than 3 movements in 8 hours

     b) Ankle edema: Dorsiflect feet frequently, avoid garters, and elevate feet as much as possible.
     c) Varicose veins: Participate in regular exercise, elevate legs, and wear support hose.
     d) Flatulence: Avoid gas-forming foods and chew thoroughly.
     e) Constipation: Drink 8–10 glasses of fluid daily, include fiber in diet, and possibly use stool softeners.
     f) Hemorrhoids: Gently push hemorrhoids inside, if possible, and avoid constipation.
     g) Leg cramps: Stretch the muscle by foot flexion and determine possible need for supplemental calcium.
     h) Faintness: Sit down and place head between legs, get to source of fresh air, and get up slowly from supine position.
     i) Shortness of breath: Sit up straight and prop up head with pillows at night.
     j) Round ligament pain: Use heating pad or bring knees up to abdomen.
     k) Insomnia: Have back massage, use effleurage, take warm shower, and drink warm milk.
  2. Instruct client in physical preparation for delivery.
     a) Present information about breastfeeding and bottle feeding.
     b) Have couple arrange for tour of birthing environment (i.e., hospital or birth center).
     c) Encourage selection of layette, diapers, and nursery equipment.
     d) Encourage selection of and participation in childbirth education classes.

3. Instruct client about signs and symptoms of labor: onset of regular contractions, loss of mucus plug, rupture of membranes.
4. Review danger signals: vaginal bleeding, swelling of face or fingers, dimmed or blurred vision, severe headache, persistent vomiting, chills, and fever.
5. Reassure client about normal discomforts of pregnancy and emphasize that the goal of good prenatal care is fetal well-being.
6. Teach client that she must wear a car safety belt, with the shoulder strap above the uterus and below the neck and the lap belt low and under the abdomen.

D. Nursing evaluation
1. Client is informed about problems that may arise and remedies for them.
2. Client has initiated physical preparation for delivery and care for the baby at home.
3. Client knows signs and symptoms of labor.
4. Client knows what danger signals need to be reported immediately.
5. Client is reassured that by following the prenatal plan of care, she is maximizing optimal maternal and fetal outcome.
6. Client understands the importance and technique of wearing a car safety belt.

See text pages

_____

VI. Nutrition during pregnancy

A. Weight gain during pregnancy
1. Normal weight gain
   a) Average overall weight gain: 24–30 lb, depending on client's height, bone structure, and prepregnancy nutritional state
   b) Pattern of weight gain
      (1) First trimester: little gain (2–4 lb), with growth mainly in maternal tissue
      (2) Second trimester: increased gain (1 lb per week), with gain mostly in maternal blood volume, fat, fluid, and enlargement of breasts and uterus
      (3) Third trimester: 1 lb per week, with gain primarily of fetus, placenta, and amniotic fluid
2. Hazards of deviations in weight gain
   a) Underweight (prepregnant weight 10% or more below standard weight for age and height): risk of low-birth-weight infant, prematurity, and pregnancy-induced hypertension (PIH)
   b) Inadequate gain (gain of 2 lb or less per month in second and third trimesters): associated with low-birth-weight infants and intrauterine growth retardation (IUGR)

c) Overweight (prepregnant weight 20% or more above standard weight for age and height): risk of gestational diabetes, large baby, hypertension, and PIH

d) Excessive gain (gain of 6.5 lb or more per month or sharp increase of 3–5 lb per week): may be indication of fluid retention and development of PIH

B. Maternal nutritional needs: increased need for almost all nutrients
  1. Recommended daily allowances (RDAs) for pregnant and lactating women: source for increased nutritional requirements
  2. Required dietary components and reasons for increase during pregnancy
    a) Calories: required for increased basal metabolic rate (BMR), for energy needs, and to allow protein to be used for tissue synthesis and maintenance rather than energy expenditure; predominantly supplied by carbohydrates (especially during last 2 trimesters)
    b) Protein: needed to provide amino acids for fetal development, blood volume expansion, and growth of maternal tissues (breasts and uterus); contributes to body's overall energy metabolism
    c) Fat: source of energy (RDA for fat is less than 30% of daily caloric intake; less than 10% should be saturated fat.)
    d) Minerals
      (1) Functions: constituents of vital body materials, with some acting as regulators and activators of body functions
      (2) Types: calcium, phosphorus, zinc, iodine, magnesium, iron, sodium
      (3) Sodium: should not be restricted (too little may damage mother and fetus), but excessive amounts should be avoided to prevent fluid retention
    e) Vitamins
      (1) Functions: involved in regulating metabolism of nutrients and assist in regulating reactions that maintain body tissues
      (2) Supplied by the diet in minute amounts and most not synthesized by the body
      (3) Types: categorized by solubility
        (a) Water-soluble: C, folic acid, B_1 (thiamin), B_2 (riboflavin), B_6 (pyridoxine) and B_{12} (cobalamin), niacin
        (b) Fat-soluble: A, D, E, K
    f) Supplementation
      (1) Ideally, diet should supply all required vitamins and minerals.
      (2) Iron and folic acid are most frequently recommended supplements because of difficulty in obtaining through diet alone (deficiency of folic acid linked to possible neural tube defects).
      (3) Excessive supplementation, especially of vitamins A and D, may have teratogenic effects on fetus.

3. Water
   a) Functions: assists digestion, aids in transport and exchanges of nutrients and wastes, and maintains body temperature
   b) Recommended consumption: 6–8 glasses of water or juices every 24 hours

C. Nutritional risk factors
   1. Prior to pregnancy
      a) 3 or more pregnancies within 2 years or 1 pregnancy that has directly progressed into another, resulting in depleted nutrient stores
      b) History of poor course or outcome of prior pregnancies, such as poor weight gain, PIH, stillbirth or low-birth-weight infant, prematurity, or perinatal infection
      c) Young maternal age, because of tendency to be underweight, to not want to gain weight, and to have poor dietary habits
      d) Economic deprivation, causing inability to purchase sufficient or nutritionally adequate food
      e) Faddish or inadequate diets
      f) Excessive use or abuse of cigarettes, alcohol, or drugs, because it interferes with adequate consumption of nutritional foods
      g) Preexisting medical condition, which may interfere with ingestion, absorption, or utilization of nutrients
         (1) Anemia, diabetes, thyroid disease
         (2) Lactose intolerance: causes increased requirements for calcium
         (3) Pica (craving to eat nonfood items): causes iron deficiency
      h) Weight problems (same as sections VI,A,2,a and VI,A,2,c of this chapter)
   2. During pregnancy
      a) Insufficient prepregnant iron stores: may require iron supplementation to meet fetal demands and to maintain hemoglobin
      b) Weight-gain problems (same as sections VI,A,2,b and VI,A,2,d of this chapter)
      c) Weight-loss problems: ketonemia, resulting in harm to fetus

D. Nutritional assessment
   1. Interview
      a) Obtain health history data from prenatal record.
         (1) Obstetric history: client's age and number, intervals, and outcomes of pregnancies

(2) Past medical history: diabetes, cystic fibrosis, anemia, lactose intolerance
    b) Identify social and environmental factors.
        (1) Home setting, socioeconomic status, family members, food assistance needs, family roles and attitudes about food
        (2) Psychologic aspects of nutrition: appetite, food choices, food associations
        (3) Religious, racial, and ethnic background
        (4) Individual dietary patterns
        (5) Psychologic conditions: anorexia, bulimia, depression
    c) Identify food allergies or intolerances.
2. Ways to determine dietary intake
    a) Questionnaire to assess client's food habits and related nutritional concerns
    b) 24-hour recall: Client writes down her food intake for past 24 hours.
    c) Food record or food diary: Client records everything eaten for 2 or 3 days.
    d) Dietary history: Client details her food intake for a typical day.
3. Physical examination
    a) Assess hair, skin, nails, muscle tone, eyes, glands, reflexes, and heart rate and rhythm for normal appearance and condition (see Nurse Alert, "Signs of Malnutrition in Pregnant Woman").
    b) Evaluate dental health status: Determine caries or periodontitis, both of which cause mechanical and mastication difficulties that interfere with ingestion.

! NURSE *ALERT* !

Signs of Malnutrition in Pregnant Woman

- Dull, dry hair; hair falling out
- Dry, flaky skin; dyspigmentation; depigmentation
- Bleeding gums, receding gums
- Missing teeth
- Swollen, raw tongue
- Enlarged thyroid gland
- Brittle, ridged nails; spoon-shaped nails
- Poor muscle tone; undeveloped, tender muscles
- Rapid heart beat, abnormal heart rhythm
- Enlarged liver or spleen
- Irritability, confusion
- Poor ankle and knee reflexes
- Listlessness, apathy

c) Conduct anthropometry.
   (1) Height and weight determination
      (a) Compare height to pregravid weight to get estimate of body build, determine standard weight, and identify underweight client.
      (b) Record weight at intervals to determine pattern of weight gain and compare with recommended pattern.
   (2) Skinfold thickness determination: assessment of relative fatness
  4. Laboratory tests
   a) Hemoglobin and hematocrit: measured routinely to evaluate iron level and need for supplements
   b) Serum folacin and B_{12}: indicate nutritional intake
   c) Serum albumin and total serum protein: if deficient, indicate predisposition to edema
   d) Glucose: urine routinely tested to screen for latent diabetes mellitus or gestational glycosuria
   e) Serum glucose: provides most accurate data about ability to utilize glucose

E. Nursing diagnoses
  1. Altered nutrition, less than body requirements, related to:
   a) Imbalance of intake versus activity expenditures
   b) Inability to procure food
   c) Chewing difficulties secondary to poor dental hygiene
   d) Poor dietary habits
  2. Knowledge deficit related to:
   a) Adequate nutrition or reliance on vitamin-mineral supplementation
   b) Weight gain and patterns during pregnancy and the specifics of her own weight gain
   c) Nutritional-related discomforts of pregnancy
   d) Cultural, ethnic, or religious influences on nutritional choices
   e) Iron and vitamin-mineral supplementation
  3. Potential for injury to fetus related to overdose of vitamins

F. Nursing intervention
  1. Discuss with client the need for increased quantity and quality of nutritional intake to support the increased energy expenditures for optimal maternal and fetal outcome.
  2. Discuss ways in which client and family can obtain assistance in food purchases (e.g., WIC program or food stamps).
  3. Schedule or refer client for dental treatment.

4. Explain to client the importance of the specific dietary components and nutritional supplements.
5. Review schedule and pattern of desirable weight gain.
6. Stress that nutritional deficiencies cannot be made up by vitamin supplementation alone.
7. Teach the basic food groups and the basic guidelines for good nutrition during pregnancy.
8. Develop sample menu plan.
9. Discuss how client's food choices related to cultural and ethnic background may need to be modified to meet increased maternal and fetal needs.
10. Teach client about increased need for iron, risk of anemia, and why iron supplementation is necessary.
11. Stress that too high an intake of vitamins can be injurious to fetal health.

G. Nursing evaluation
1. Client understands the importance of good nutrition during pregnancy, the specific requirements, and how to include them in meal planning.
2. Client is able to identify sources of food at reduced costs.
3. Client receives dental care, if necessary.
4. Client understands the amount of weight she can gain and the pattern of gain throughout her pregnancy.
5. Client is aware of the need for supplementation with iron, vitamins, and minerals but that there is a danger to the fetus of excess supplementation.
6. Client understands how to modify food choices based on cultural or ethnic background, if necessary.

VII. Preparation for childbirth

A. Methods of prepared childbirth
1. Grantly Dick-Read method or psychophysical preparation: Focus is on replacing fear of the unknown with understanding and confidence.
   a) Program components
      (1) Education to help clients comprehend the physiologic processes of labor
      (2) Exercises to improve muscle tone and to foster relaxation
      (3) Breathing patterns to use during stages of labor: combination of deep abdominal respirations, shallow breaths from diaphragm, and panting breaths
   b) Advantages
      (1) Baby may be healthier because of reduced need for analgesics and anesthetics.
      (2) Childbirth can be shared by couple.

See text pages
_____

2. Lamaze method (also known as psychoprophylactic method): Focus is on the client developing a conditioned response not to experience pain in labor.
   a) Program components
      (1) Education on exercises, breathing techniques, and theories of learning and motivation
      (2) Relaxation exercises to achieve active involvement of mind over body (e.g., progressive relaxation, touch relaxation, disassociation relaxation)
      (3) Use of imagery in which a person focuses concentration on one object to decrease pain
      (4) Breathing techniques to keep pressure of the diaphragm off the contracting uterus; performed during labor to help client control pain; choice of types by client depends on effectiveness, not on stage of labor
         (a) Cleansing breath (done at the start and end of each contraction): inhalation through nose and exhalation through pursed lips
         (b) Slow, deep breathing (also called slow-paced breathing) in which client inhales through nose (moving only her chest) and exhales through pursed lips
         (c) Shallow breathing (also called modified-paced breathing) in which client inhales and exhales at rate of 4–5 breaths every 5 seconds
         (d) Pant-blow breathing (also called pattern-paced breathing): similar to rapid shallow breathing except for the use of forceful exhalation through pursed lips after every few breaths
   b) Advantages
      (1) Client has more control over the management of pain during contractions.
      (2) Expanded educational component now covers nutrition, infant feeding, cesarean birth, sexuality, early parenting, and coping skills.
3. Bradley method (also known as husband-coached childbirth): Focus is on use of labor breathing techniques, the husband as "coach," and modifications of the environment.
   a) Program components
      (1) Slow, deep, abdominal breathing and general body relaxation
      (2) Use of darkness, solitude, and quiet to make childbirth a more natural experience
   b) Advantages: discourages the use of any medication

4. Cesarean birth: Focus is on treating cesarean birth as a normal event.
   a) Program components: presentation of factual information about what will happen, use and effects of regional anesthesia, what the couple will feel, and in what ways they can participate
   b) Advantages: diminishes fear of unknown and prepares couple for possibility of cesarean birth

B. Birthing environments
   1. Hospital setting
      a) Traditional labor and delivery room with sterile procedures and usually little choice in birthing position
      b) Trend toward labor-delivery-recovery (LDR) rooms and/or labor-delivery-recovery-postpartum (LDRP) rooms with homelike accommodations and technology available if needed
   2. Freestanding birth center
      a) Separate from but close to hospital facilities, with policies about when to transfer client to hospital
      b) Physicians with staff privileges at local hospital and certified nurse-midwives in attendance
      c) Birthing rooms similar to typical bedrooms
      d) Selection by the family of a birth plan that outlines the practices and procedures members would like included or excluded
   3. Home birth
      a) Chance for delivery in a familiar setting
      b) Difficulty in providing backup care for labor emergencies: possible reluctance by physicians to arrange emergency backup in advance
      c) Difficulty finding qualified medical personnel to attend delivery
      d) Not a safe choice for high-risk pregnancy

C. Childbirth classes
   1. Early classes (first trimester): emphasis on early gestational changes, self-care during pregnancy, fetal development, sexuality during pregnancy, nutrition, rest and exercises, psychologic changes in pregnancy, relief measures for discomfort
   2. Later classes (second and third trimesters): preparation for birth process, postpartum self-care, birth choices, newborn safety issues, breastfeeding programs

D. Family involvement
   1. Sibling preparation: Birth of a new sibling may be associated with negative behavior, but inclusion (e.g., tour of maternity ward, discussion of birth process, and discussion of what babies are like) may increase developmental maturity.
   2. Grandparent preparation: They can be important sources of support and information for prospective and new parents. Inclusion in preparation process may increase family support.

E. Essential nursing care
  1. Nursing assessment
      a) Assess the couple's information base and need for additional information.
      b) Identify who will accompany the client in labor, what the birthing choice is, and where the couple would like the birth to occur.
      c) Ascertain the cultural or ethnic variations the couple would like to honor during the birthing process.
      d) Identify the mother's preferences regarding analgesia, enema, perineal preparation, and birth position.
  2. Nursing diagnoses
      a) Knowledge deficit related to information needs during pregnancy and childbirth
      b) Knowledge deficit related to self-care measures during childbirth
      c) Ineffective individual coping related to unknown childbirth environment
      d) Altered family processes related to the arrival of an additional member
  3. Nursing intervention
      a) Inform the couple about the different childbirth methods and settings in which childbirth can occur.
      b) Teach the specific self-care techniques that the couple prefer to use during labor and delivery, or refer the couple to appropriate classes.
      c) Help the couple select the most appropriate birthing technique for them.
      d) Assist the couple in selecting the appropriate childbirth class.
      e) Reassure the couple that they will have sufficient information and skills to have the optimum birth experience.
      f) Teach the couple how other family members can participate in the birthing experience.
  4. Nursing evaluation
      a) The couple understand the different methods and environments from which they can choose.
      b) The couple learn the relaxation and breathing techniques that they will use during childbirth.
      c) The couple have enrolled in a childbirth class that focuses on their particular needs.
      d) The couple are less anxious about the childbirth process and feel more able to have a satisfying experience.
      e) Siblings and grandparents are more knowledgeable about the birth and are able to participate and/or be supportive.

1. Mrs. Adams is expecting her third child. Her other children, both born at term, are ages 2 and 5. Mrs. Adams has had an abortion. Mrs. Adams's gravida/para status is:

   a. gravida 2, para 2102.
   b. gravida 4, para 2012.
   c. gravida 3, para 2012.
   d. gravida 3, para 2002.

2. At her first prenatal visit, Mrs. Adams tells the nurse that the first day of her last menstrual period (LMP) was December 15, 1993. Using Nägele's rule for determining the estimated date of birth (EDB), the correct date should be:

   a. August 22, 1994.
   b. September 8, 1994.
   c. September 22, 1994.
   d. October 15, 1994.

3. While doing the vaginal examination on Mrs. Adams, the nurse notes that the cervix has a bluish color. This is known as:

   a. Hegar's sign.
   b. Goodell's sign.
   c. Ballottement.
   d. Chadwick's sign.

4. Which piece of data obtained from Mrs. Adams during the initial interview would put Mrs. Adams at risk during her pregnancy?

   a. Rubella at age 10
   b. Tetanus toxoid vaccine (perhaps after conception)
   c. Smoker (1 pack of cigarettes a day)
   d. Previous abortion (no complications)

5. At each prenatal visit, Mrs. Adams can expect to have:

   a. Hemoglobin and hematocrit.
   b. Urine cultures.
   c. Ultrasonography.
   d. Fundal height measurements.

6. While assessing a client, the nurse would identify which of the following manifestations as a probable sign of pregnancy?

   a. Absence of menstruation
   b. Nausea and vomiting
   c. Enlargement of the abdomen and uterus
   d. Breast tenderness and fullness

7. Kari, age 15, is 28 weeks pregnant. During a routine prenatal visit, the nurse assesses that Kari's skin is dry and itchy. Kari states that she tires easily and is often irritable. Her weight at last month's visit was 121 lb and today is 122 lb. Her hemoglobin is 10.2 g/dl. Kari states, "I'm just not interested in eating." Based on the assessment data, the most appropriate nursing diagnosis for Kari is:

   a. Knowledge deficit related to nutritional needs during pregnancy.
   b. Fatigue related to pregnancy.
   c. Altered nutrition, less than body requirements, related to anorexia.
   d. Altered nutrition, less than body requirements, related to self-imposed calorie restrictions.

8. Kari tells the nurse that she doesn't drink milk and doesn't like meat. Alternative protein-rich foods that the nurse could suggest for Kari are:

   a. Peanut butter, cooked dry beans, and yogurt.
   b. Cottage cheese, cooked cereal, and oranges.
   c. Pasta, tomatoes, and salads.
   d. Beans, broccoli, and cheese.

9. When Kari returns to the clinic the following month, the best indicator that Kari is meeting nutritional goals is:

   a. Fetal heart tones, 152 bpm.
   b. Weight gain of 3 lb.
   c. Blood pressure, 108/68.
   d. Urine glucose, negative.

10. During a prenatal visit, the Dixons ask the nurse about the value of childbirth education classes. The nurse explains that the goal of the classes is to:

   a. Equip a couple for pain-free childbirth.
   b. Provide a couple with knowledge and skills to actively participate in labor and delivery.
   c. Eliminate anxiety in order to have an uncomplicated birth.
   d. Empower a couple to totally control the labor and delivery process.

11. Janice is 32 weeks pregnant. During a prenatal visit, she tells the nurse that she often feels faint and dizzy when she lies on her back. The physiologic rationale for these symptoms is:

   a. Supine hypotension.
   b. Anemia.
   c. Dehydration.
   d. Infection.

12. While completing a vaginal exam on Mrs. Perletti, the nurse notes that the client has poor muscle tone of the pubococcygeal muscle. The nurse should:

   a. Encourage partial sit-ups.
   b. Teach Kegel exercises.
   c. Demonstrate pelvic tilt exercises.
   d. Encourage a "tailor sit" position.

ANSWERS

1. **Correct answer is b.**

   • The gravida number refers to the number of pregnancies including the current one. For Mrs. Adams, this number is 4.
   • Para refers to the number of births/deliveries. The first digit represents the total number of term deliveries. For Mrs. Adams, this number is 2.
   • The second digit refers to the number of preterm babies. For Mrs. Adams, this number is 0.
   • The third digit refers to the number of abortions. For Mrs. Adams, this number is 1.
   • The fourth digit refers to number of living children. For Mrs. Adams, this number is 2.
   a, c, and **d.** All are incorrect based on the data given in correct answer b.

2. **Correct answer is c.** Nägele's rule is: Add 7 days to the first day of the last menstrual period, subtract 3 months, and add 1 year (if necessary). Nägele's rule assumes a 28-day menstrual cycle. Adjustments may be necessary for shorter or longer cycles.

   a, b, and **d.** All are incorrect based on Nägele's rule.

3. **Correct answer is d.** Discoloration of the cervix is known as Chadwick's sign. This occurs during the early weeks of pregnancy when there is increased blood flow to the uterus.

   a. Hegar's sign is a softening of the lower part of the uterus that occurs at 6–8 weeks of pregnancy.
   b. Goodell's sign is the softening of the cervix that occurs in early pregnancy.
   c. Ballottement is a technique of detecting passive movements of the unengaged fetus as it floats in amniotic fluid.

4. **Correct answer is c.** Smoking is significant for future prenatal care since maternal smoking has a negative impact on the fetus (e.g., fetal growth retardation and preterm labor). The nurse needs to counsel Mrs. Adams to quit smoking or at least cut back.

   a. History of rubella is not a risk factor. Mrs. Adams will have rubella titer drawn to verify antibodies.
   b. Receiving a tetanus toxoid vaccine is not contraindicated during pregnancy.
   d. History of previous abortion is not a risk factor unless there were complications.

5. **Correct answer is d.** Fundal height is measured during each prenatal visit. Height of the fundus can be used as an indicator of fetal growth and as an estimator of gestational age.

a. Hemoglobin and hematocrit are done at the first prenatal visit and at 30–32 weeks to detect anemia. They are not a routine part of each visit unless signs and symptoms warrant them.
b. Urine cultures are done when signs and symptoms of possible urinary tract infection are present.
c. Ultrasonography is not to be expected at each prenatal visit. It may be done to determine fetal age between 8 and 16 weeks and again as indicated during pregnancy.

6. **Correct answer is c.** Enlargement of the abdomen and uterus during the childbearing years is regarded as a probable sign of pregnancy.

a and b. Absence of menstruation and nausea and vomiting may result from a number of conditions other than pregnancy. Menstrual suppression and nausea and vomiting are presumptive signs of pregnancy.
d. Breast tenderness and fullness are noted by many women prior to the menstrual period. The early breast changes associated with pregnancy are a presumptive sign of pregnancy.

7. **Correct answer is c.** Appropriate nursing diagnosis is based on data presented (signs of malnutrition) and is related to the fact that Kari is disinterested in eating.

a. There are no data here to support a knowledge deficit.
b. Kari's fatigue is a symptom of inadequate nutritional intake, especially during the second trimester.
d. There are no data presented that indicate that Kari is deliberately imposing a restricted diet on herself. Rather, she is anorexic and has no appetite.

8. **Correct answer is a.** All of these foods are protein-rich. In addition, vegetable protein will also supply folic acid and fiber. Yogurt supplies calcium.

b. Cottage cheese provides protein and calcium. However, neither cooked cereal nor oranges are considered protein-rich.
c. Pasta provides carbohydrates as well as vitamins but is not protein-rich. Salads and tomatoes are also excellent sources of vitamins and minerals but are not high in protein.
d. Although beans and cheese supply protein, broccoli does not. However, broccoli is a good source of vitamins.

9. **Correct answer is b.** A weight gain reflects improved nutritional intake for Kari. She is almost at the accepted norm of 1 lb per week during the second trimester.

a. These are normal fetal heart tones and do not necessarily represent nutritional intake.
c. This blood pressure reading does not reflect nutritional intake and is within normal BP readings.
d. A negative urine glucose is normal. A small degree of glycosuria may be present in pregnancy but reflects kidney filtration, not necessarily nutritional intake.

10. **Correct answer is b.** Childbirth education classes present information regarding the labor and delivery process, as well as specific skills such as breathing techniques, that enhances a couple's participation in labor and delivery.

a. No childbirth education class can equip a couple for pain-free childbirth. Classes do prepare individuals for ways to respond to pain and teach techniques to decrease the pain experience.
c. Women do experience anxiety during labor and delivery. Anxiety is not a predictor for complications of birth.
d. No couple can totally control the labor and delivery process. Some variables are out of their control (e.g., presentation of the fetus).

11. **Correct answer is a.** The enlarging uterus may cause pressure on the vena cava when a woman lies supine. This causes a marked decrease in blood pressure with symptoms of dizziness, pallor, and clamminess. It is corrected by assuming a left side-lying position.

b. Symptoms of anemia are fatigue and pallor.
c. Some symptoms of dehydration are fatigue, weakness, and dry mucous membranes.
d. Symptoms of infection are urinary frequency, chills, and fever.

12. **Correct answer is b.** Perineal muscle tightening, also known as Kegel exercises, strengthens the pubococcygeal muscle and increases its elasticity. Firmness of the muscle improves support to the pelvic organs.

a. Partial abdominal sit-ups are encouraged to tighten the abdominal muscles.
c. Pelvic tilt exercises are done to prevent or reduce back strain and strengthen abdominal muscle tone.
d. Assuming a "tailor sit" position stretches the muscles of the inner thighs in preparation for labor and birth.

6

High-Risk Conditions and Complications during Pregnancy

NURSING HIGHLIGHTS

1. Nurse should be nonjudgmental, concrete, and realistic throughout care of high-risk clients.
2. Medical illnesses, such as heart disease, diabetes, and hypertension, may be stressed by the pregnant state but usually can be managed if treatment is initiated early and progress monitored closely.

3. Nurse should educate high-risk client about danger signals that warn of problems in the pregnancy and should emphasize need for immediate care.
4. The goal in premature rupture of membranes and preterm labor is to delay delivery as long as possible to allow for fetal lung maturity.
5. Nurse should provide ongoing reassurance and information during prenatal diagnostic testing procedures to help reduce anxiety levels of client.
6. Nurse should provide education to clients about teratogenic agents that can harm fetal development.

GLOSSARY

cephalopelvic disproportion (CPD)—condition in which fetal head is too large for passage through maternal pelvis

clonus—series of rapid, rhythmic, involuntary muscle contractions occurring as a result of stretching muscle

complete abortion—abortion in which all products of conception have been passed

Couvelaire uterus—excessive bleeding into uterine muscle because of abruptio placentae

habitual abortion—spontaneous abortion occurring in 3 or more consecutive pregnancies

incomplete abortion—abortion in which only some products of conception are passed

missed abortion—condition in which fetus has died but products of conception remain in uterus

polyhydramnios—excessive amount of amniotic fluid, usually more than 2000 ml

ENHANCED OUTLINE

See text pages
_____

I. Preexisting maternal physical conditions

A. Age (<16 or >35)
   1. Adolescent pregnancy (<16 years)
      a) Physiologic risks (related to lack of early prenatal care, early gynecological age, poor nutrition, smoking, and substance abuse): low-birth-weight infants, pregnancy-induced hypertension (PIH), iron deficiency anemia, cephalopelvic disproportion (CPD), sexually transmitted diseases (STDs), stillbirth or prematurity, dystocia

b) Psychosocial risks (related to underdeveloped developmental skills, especially in younger adolescents): poor body image, extended dependence on parents, inability to develop relationships with peers, low economic and social stability

c) Nursing assessment (see sections IV, V, and VI of Chapter 5 for details of assessment of pregnant woman)

    (1) Special concerns in obtaining adolescent's history: past history of STDs; use of caffeine, nicotine, alcohol, and over-the-counter and recreational drugs; dietary history and nutritional status; immunization history; sexual history

    (2) Special issues in physical examination and lab testing

        (a) Baseline weight

        (b) Blood pressure

        (c) Hematocrit and hemoglobin

        (d) Cultures for various STDs

        (e) Pelvic exam: clinical pelvimetry to determine spatial capacity and risk for CPD; cervical cytology and culture

    (3) Special concerns in assessing cognitive and psychosocial readiness: adolescent's developmental level, family support level, financial support system, ability to do self-evaluation

d) Nursing diagnoses

    (1) Knowledge deficit related to:

        (a) Fetal growth and development

        (b) Nutritional needs of pregnancy

        (c) Self-care

    (2) Altered nutrition: less than (or more than) body requirements related to poor dietary habits

    (3) Body image disturbance related to weight gain and altered body dimensions

    (4) High risk for altered parenting related to impaired parent-infant attachment and adolescent egocentrism

e) Nursing intervention

    (1) Explain normal fetal growth and development and the importance of regularly scheduled assessment of the client and fetus.

    (2) Discuss relationship between weight gain, dietary intake, and fetal development; help determine nutritious diet.

    (3) Counsel client about normal body changes and ways to promote positive self-image.

    (4) Discuss parenting skills and infant care; refer client and father (if available) to childbirth preparation and parenting classes.

f) Nursing evaluation

    (1) Client understands the normal process of pregnancy and attends scheduled prenatal visits.

    (2) Client understands the importance of a balanced diet and selects food to meet those needs, reflected by recommended weight gain.

(3) Client feels more comfortable with her changing body and sees herself in a more positive light.

(4) Client understands parenting responsibilities and plans to attend childbirth preparation and parenting classes.

(5) Client utilizes available resources to assist meeting her physiologic, psychosocial, and financial needs.

2. Pregnancy in women over 35

   a) Physiologic risks: PIH, gestational diabetes, placenta previa, malpresentation, premature labor, dystocia, postpartum hemorrhage due to presence of fibroids; fetus at greater risk for Down syndrome or other chromosomal abnormalities; possible need for cesarean birth

   b) Psychosocial concerns: worry over parental energy level, social isolation, attitude of family members

   c) Nursing assessment (see sections IV, V, and VI of Chapter 5 for details of assessment of pregnant woman): special attention to possible use of amniocentesis or chorionic villus sampling to detect chromosomal abnormalities

   d) Nursing diagnoses

      (1) Knowledge deficit related to specific risks of pregnancy over 35

      (2) Altered family processes related to pregnancy changes

      (3) Family coping: potential for growth related to tasks of pregnancy

      (4) Potential for decisional conflict related to continuing pregnancy

   e) Nursing intervention

      (1) Identify and explain to client possible health risks.

      (2) Promote adaptation to pregnancy including the adjustments to be made by other family members.

      (3) Provide support regarding diagnostic testing and decision couple may have to make.

      (4) Recommend genetic counseling, if appropriate.

   f) Nursing evaluation

      (1) Client is knowledgeable about her pregnancy, the risks for the fetus, and testing that may be required.

      (2) Client adapts to and copes with pregnancy.

      (3) Client receives adequate prenatal care.

B. Heart disease

  1. Preexisting types: rheumatic heart disease, congenital heart defects, valvular dysfunction (mitral valve prolapse)

2. Pregnancy-onset type: peripartum cardiomyopathy (dysfunction of left ventricle in last month of pregnancy or early postpartum period)
3. Risks imposed by pregnancy (see Chapter 5, section I,F, for effect of pregnancy on normal cardiovascular system)
   a) Maternal: cardiac decompensation and congestive heart failure (caused by increased blood volume of pregnancy), PIH, clotting disorder, side effects of tocolytic therapy
   b) Fetal/neonatal: fetal and infant morbidity and mortality, prematurity, low birth weight
4. Medical therapy
   a) Goal is early diagnosis and initiation of treatment.
   b) Therapy is monitored using classification system, based on client's functional capacity: Class I (no limitation of physical activity) to Class IV (inability to carry on any physical activity without experiencing pain).
   c) Regimen may include antibiotics, anticoagulants, diuretics, digitalis, antiarrhythmic agents, changing tocolytic agents.
5. Nursing assessment
   a) Obtain medical history, assess functional capacity and activity level, observe for signs of cardiac decompensation (cough, dyspnea, edema, heart murmurs, palpitations, rales).
   b) Identify other cardiac stress factors: anemia, weight gain, infection.
   c) Monitor heart sounds and screen for signs of PIH.
6. Nursing diagnoses
   a) Activity intolerance related to increased metabolic requirements of pregnancy
   b) Decreased cardiac output and circulation related to physiologic demands of pregnancy
   c) Impaired gas exchange related to pulmonary edema
   d) Knowledge deficit related to:
      (1) Signs and symptoms of complications of cardiac conditions
      (2) Self-care activities
      (3) Effects of cardiac condition on pregnancy
   e) Anxiety related to fears concerning perinatal outcome
7. Nursing intervention
   a) Teach client about need to reduce stress, increase rest, modify activity levels, and avoid contact with infected people.
   b) Teach client about changes in cardiac function and alterations that need to be made.
      (1) Diet high in iron, protein, and vitamins but low in salt
      (2) Prenatal visits every 2 weeks for the first half of pregnancy and then weekly
      (3) Special intrapartal considerations (e.g., use of analgesics during labor to reduce discomfort and anxiety)
   c) Inform client of symptoms of cardiac decompensation and other complications.

        d) Review prescribed medications with client to clarify action and detect possible side effects.

        e) Monitor client at frequent intervals and immediately report changes in cardiac status.

    8. Nursing evaluation

        a) Client understands the mechanisms of cardiac function and alterations that may occur during her pregnancy.

        b) Client does what she can to prevent complications.

        c) Client can identify signs and symptoms of cardiac decompensation and other complications.

        d) Client understands special labor and delivery considerations caused by her condition.

        e) Client has realistic view of her physiologic status and possible outcome for fetus.

C. Diabetes mellitus

    1. Types

        a) Preexisting: type I, insulin-dependent; type II, not insulin-dependent; impaired glucose tolerance

        b) Gestational diabetes (pregnancy-induced)

    2. Risks imposed by pregnancy (see Chapter 5, section I,L,6, for effect of pregnancy on normal pancreas, which produces insulin)

        a) Maternal: PIH, preeclampsia, hydramnios, macrosomia, large placenta, ketoacidosis, dystocia, anemia, infection, cesarean delivery

        b) Fetal/neonatal: congenital abnormalities, hypoglycemia, hypocalcemia, prematurity, respiratory distress syndrome, large for gestational age (LGA), spontaneous abortion, intrauterine growth retardation (IUGR), small for gestational age (SGA), hyperbilirubinemia, macrosomia, fetal and neonatal mortality (see also Chapter 10, section I,A)

    3. Medical therapy

        a) Identification of at-risk client: screening tests and glucose tolerance tests

        b) Early prenatal care

        c) Prevention, detection, and control of complications through:

            (1) Glucose monitoring (daily, in many cases)

            (2) Ultrasound

            (3) Nonstress test

        d) Management of glucose levels by combination of insulin, diet, and exercise (need for insulin will increase throughout pregnancy)

4. Nursing assessment
   a) Obtain pertinent history of previous large infant, family history, unexplained stillborn, prior delivery of infant with congenital anomaly, maternal obesity, hypertension, glycosuria, recurrent urinary tract infection or vaginitis, large or poor weight gain in pregnancy, and presence of polyhydramnios.
   b) Perform physical exam including fundoscopy and palpation for polyhydramnios or large fetus.
   c) Order laboratory tests including glycosylated hemoglobin, blood glucose, and urine testing for glucose and ketones.
   d) Ascertain client's ability to cope with stress of pregnancy and diabetes and to follow regimen of care.
5. Nursing diagnoses
   a) Knowledge deficit related to:
      (1) Diabetes and prognosis
      (2) Effects of insulin and its administration
      (3) Diabetic self-care measures
      (4) Nutrition needs of pregnancy
   b) Self-concept disturbances related to loss of control over self-care
   c) Fear related to complications of pregnancy
   d) High risk for infection and injury related to poor control of blood glucose
6. Nursing intervention
   a) Explain pathophysiology of diabetes and its effects on client and fetus.
   b) If client is insulin-dependent, explain the effects of insulin, how it is administered, and the reason for probable dosage changes as pregnancy progresses.
   c) Teach client home blood glucose monitoring and signs, symptoms, and treatment of hypoglycemia.
   d) Identify for client a proper diet (2200–2500 calories) and the importance of having carbohydrates be 45% of total.
   e) Promote use of planned program of physical exercise.
   f) Provide supportive care to client regarding the impact of diagnosis on pregnancy.
   g) Teach client the importance of early intervention for signs of infection or other complications of pregnancy.
   h) Monitor client at frequent intervals and immediately report abnormal glucose levels or changes in fetal heart rate or fetal activity pattern.
7. Nursing evaluation
   a) Client understands her disease and its treatment.
   b) Client is reassured that early identification of problems and compliance with treatment plan increase safety for herself and the fetus.
   c) Client's blood glucose remains in optimal range (60–120 mg/dl).

D. Iron deficiency anemia: hemoglobin below 10–11 g/dl; hematocrit less than 33%–35%
   1. Risks during pregnancy
      a) Maternal: susceptibility to infection, fatigue, increased chance of PIH and postpartum hemorrhage, cardiac failure
      b) Fetal/neonatal: low birth weight, prematurity, small for gestational age, stillbirth
   2. Medical therapy: prophylactic iron supplementation, preferably oral
   3. Nursing assessment: Examine for pallor of skin and conjunctivae and for fatigue; obtain complete blood count.
   4. Nursing diagnoses
      a) Altered nutrition, less than body requirements for iron, related to poor intake of iron-rich foods
      b) High risk for constipation related to iron intake
   5. Nursing intervention: Provide daily iron (300 mg ferrous sulfate) with orange juice; review dietary elements rich in iron; recommend stool softeners.
   6. Nursing evaluation
      a) Client understands the risks associated with iron deficiency anemia during pregnancy.
      b) Client takes recommended iron supplements and follows diet rich in iron.
      c) Client maintains adequate hemoglobin levels during pregnancy.

E. AIDS (acquired immunodeficiency syndrome)
   1. Risks during pregnancy
      a) Maternal: acceleration of clinical symptoms in HIV-positive, asymptomatic clients; infection
      b) Fetal/neonatal: 30%–50% risk of transmission through placenta, during passage through birth canal, in breast milk
   2. Medical therapy: treatment of opportunistic infections; no known cure but new drugs, such as AZT, show clinical promise of slowing down progression of disease
   3. Nursing assessment
      a) Identify and screen high-risk clients: prostitutes, history of STD, IV drug user, partner in high-risk categories.
      b) Identify signs and symptoms through physical exam and diagnostic tests.
   4. Nursing diagnoses
      a) Knowledge deficit related to AIDS and implications for newborn
      b) High risk for infection related to altered immunity
      c) Altered nutrition, less than body requirements, related to poor intake

      d) High risk for ineffective family coping related to lack of support system

      e) Fear related to course of disease

  5. Nursing intervention

      a) Educate client about her disease and its possible effects on her baby.

      b) Educate client about signs and symptoms of infection and the importance of notifying her physician if any of these occur.

      c) Recommend diet and educate about nutritional needs.

      d) Provide emotional support to client and her family, and recommend resources to assist with finances or counseling.

      e) Educate client about ways to prevent spread of AIDS.

  6. Nursing evaluation

      a) Client is informed about her illness, what signs to watch for, and the potential outcomes for her child.

      b) Client and family are able to verbalize their concerns and obtain additional assistance.

      c) Client knows and practices methods of preventing spread of AIDS.

F. TORCH infections

  1. TORCH: group of infections that cause the most harm to embryo and fetus: *to*xoplasmosis, *r*ubella, *c*ytomegalovirus, *h*erpes simplex virus (*O* may stand for *o*ther infections [e.g., hepatitis B, chlamydia, syphilis])

  2. Fetal/neonatal risks: prematurity, mild to severe congenital abnormalities (which may not be recognized until childhood), neonatal death

  3. Medical therapy: identification of high-risk clients, prevention, urine and serologic testing, cervical cultures, treatment if possible (no treatment for cytomegalovirus), possible counseling about therapeutic abortion

  4. Nursing assessment

      a) Identify high-risk clients.

      b) Take history of exposure or prior illness.

      c) Assess symptoms, if present.

  5. Nursing diagnoses

      a) Knowledge deficit related to impact of infection

      b) Altered health maintenance related to lack of knowledge

      c) Fear related to potential effects on fetus

      d) Potential ineffective individual coping related to depression

  6. Nursing intervention

      a) Teach client about danger of exposure and possible consequences of fetal infection.

      b) Provide emotional support to client and family about the possible fetal outcomes.

      c) Teach client about treatment methods for specific infections, if available.

7. Nursing evaluation
   a) Client understands about current or potential risk of infection and is able to identify symptoms.
   b) Client institutes health measures to avoid infection.
   c) Client expresses satisfaction regarding decision to continue or terminate pregnancy.

G. Chronic hypertensive disease: blood pressure of 140/90 mm Hg or higher before pregnancy, before 20th week of pregnancy (in absence of trophoblastic disease), or indefinitely after delivery
   1. Risks during pregnancy: development of preeclampsia and fetal and maternal mortality
   2. Medical therapy: antihypertensive and diuretic drugs, early and frequent prenatal visits, evaluation of baseline tests and routine laboratory evaluations, ultrasound, bed rest, low-protein diet, and self-monitoring of blood pressure
   3. Essential nursing care: to educate client about plan of care and how to assess fetal movement daily during rest periods

II. Gestational problems

See text pages

A. Pregnancy-induced hypertension (PIH): syndrome of hypertension, edema, and proteinuria appearing after 20th week of pregnancy
   1. Types
      a) Mild preeclampsia: early stages of PIH
      b) Severe preeclampsia
      c) HELLP (*h*emolysis, *e*levated *l*iver enzymes, *l*ow *p*latelet count) syndrome: multiple organ failure
      d) Eclampsia: severe preeclampsia that has progressed to convulsions
   2. Signs and symptoms
      a) Mild preeclampsia
         (1) Gradual or sudden increase in blood pressure of 30 mm Hg systolic or 15 mm Hg diastolic above baseline on at least 2 occasions 6 hours or more apart
         (2) Edema, causing sudden excessive weight gain (more than 1 lb/week)
         (3) Protein in urine: <5 g/l/24 hours (1–2+ on dipstick)
      b) Severe preeclampsia
         (1) Elevated blood pressure of 160/110 or higher on 2 occasions at least 6 hours apart while client is on bed rest
         (2) Protein in urine: ≥5 g/l/24 hours (3–4+ on dipstick)
         (3) Oliguria: urine output ≤400 ml/24 hours
         (4) Headache, blurred vision, scotomata

      (5) Hyperreflexia

      (6) Retinal edema

      (7) Possible progression to HELLP syndrome, requiring client to give birth promptly regardless of gestational age

   c) HELLP syndrome: includes all signs and symptoms of severe preeclampsia plus:

      (1) Hemolysis

      (2) Elevated liver enzymes

      (3) Low platelet count

   d) Eclampsia

      (1) Convulsions, possibly preceded by high temperature

      (2) Coma

      (3) Hypertensive crisis or shock

3. Additional risks: maternal mortality, disseminated intravascular coagulation, prematurity, small-for-gestational-age fetus, stillbirth

4. Medical therapy

   a) Activity restriction: may include bed rest (lying on side) and sedation

   b) Well-balanced diet with adequate protein, moderate sodium

   c) Prevention of eclamptic seizures with magnesium sulfate (MgSO$_4$) and treatment of severe hypertension with antihypertensives

   d) Evaluation of fetal status (nonstress test, biophysical profile, serial sonograms, contraction stress test)

   e) Delivery of baby if uterine environment compromised

   f) Monitoring lab values to assess vascular volume, renal and liver function, coagulation status

5. Nursing assessment

   a) Monitor maternal blood pressure, temperature, weight, and respirations.

   b) Assess fetal heart rate pattern with electronic fetal monitor to detect possible onset of distress.

   c) Assess deep tendon reflexes.

   d) Observe for pitting edema, severe headache, visual disturbances, vaginal bleeding, and abdominal tenderness.

   e) Observe for changes in level of consciousness such as irritability, disturbance in attention span, and signs of convulsion.

   f) Monitor urine output and test urine for protein and for specific gravity.

   g) Assess lab values for baseline values and changes (e.g., blood urea nitrogen (BUN), liver enzymes, blood and platelet counts).

6. Nursing diagnoses

   a) Mild PIH

      (1) Knowledge deficit related to preeclampsia and its effects on client and fetus and its management

      (2) Altered tissue perfusion (cerebral, cardiac, uteroplacental) related to vasoconstrictive effects of PIH

      (3) Ineffective individual/family coping related to client's restricted activity

b) Severe PIH
  (1) High risk for injury to client related to possibility of convulsion or effects of HELLP syndrome
  (2) High risk for injury to fetus related to inadequate placental perfusion

7. Nursing intervention
   a) Teach client pathophysiology of PIH and the signs and symptoms of preeclampsia and eclampsia.
   b) Explain to client the reasons for bed rest, and devise schedule to reduce maternal activity to increase uteroplacental perfusion.
   c) Help family cope with the changes caused if client is hospitalized.
   d) Monitor client at frequent intervals and immediately report worsening of PIH.
   e) Monitor for signs of $MgSO_4$ toxicity (see Nurse Alert, "Observing for Signs of $MgSO_4$ Toxicity").
   f) Provide ongoing supportive care to client, including safety precautions in case of convulsion or $MgSO_4$ toxicity.
   g) If labor occurs, keep client lying on side and monitor for complications (e.g., fetal distress, placental separation, renal failure).

8. Nursing evaluation
   a) Client understands PIH and can identify signs of preeclampsia and possible complications.
   b) Client follows treatment plan, including bed rest.
   c) Client does not have any eclamptic convulsions.
   d) Client delivers healthy infant.

B. Incompetent cervical os: premature dilatation of cervix (usually in 16th to 20th week)
   1. Signs and symptoms: painless dilatation, bloody show, premature rupture of membranes (PROM)
   2. Risks: late habitual abortion and preterm labor
   3. Medical therapy: cervical cerclage (allowing 80%–90% of women to carry fetus to term)
      a) Shirodkar-Barter technique: reinforcement of weakened cervix with a purse-string suture at internal os
      b) McDonald technique: use of purse-string suture on cervical mucosa
   4. Nursing assessment: Obtain history (positive history of repeated, painless, and bloodless second-trimester abortions is indicative of this condition).
   5. Nursing diagnoses
      a) Knowledge deficit related to anatomical defect
      b) Fear related to possible loss of fetus

Observing for Signs of MgSO₄ Toxicity

Client should never be left unattended.

Possible early side effects to note in client:
- Feeling of warmth
- Nausea
- Flushing
- Slurred speech
- Muscle weakness

Monitor for the following indications of toxicity:
- Hypotension: drop in blood pressure (during administration of drug or thereafter)
- Decrease in urinary output: volume under 100 ml/4 hours
- Slowing of respirations: fewer than 12–14/minute
- Serum levels of magnesium above 10 mg/dl
- Depression or absence of reflexes, especially disappearance of patella tendon reflex (knee jerk)
- Central nervous system depression: anxiety, drowsiness, lethargy
- Sudden decrease in fetal heart rate
- Cardiac arrest

Treatment:
- Discontinue use of MgSO₄.
- Keep calcium gluconate at bedside.
- Administer intravenously over 3 minutes for MgSO₄ toxicity.
- Provide oxygen via face mask at 10–12 l/minute.

6. Nursing intervention
   a) Reassure client about potential for good outcome if condition is treated appropriately.
   b) While client is on bed rest for 24 hours after cerclage, monitor for vaginal bleeding, onset of labor, and PROM.
7. Nursing evaluation
   a) Client understands the need for bed rest for at least 24 hours after procedure.
   b) Client understands that suture will stay in place until delivery.

C. Bleeding (hemorrhagic) problems in early pregnancy
   1. Spontaneous abortion: naturally occurring expulsion of fetus prior to viability (20–24 weeks)
      a) Often associated with embryonic or trophoblastic defect
      b) Signs and symptoms: pelvic cramping, bleeding, backache

       c) Medical therapy

          (1) Diagnostic findings: ultrasound showing presence of gestational sac, lowered human chorionic gonadotropin (hCG) level after fetal death, urine negative or weakly positive for hCG

          (2) For threatened abortion, bed rest and abstinence from coitus and orgasm

          (3) Blood transfusions as required

          (4) Dilatation and curettage (to remove retained products of conception)

       d) Nursing assessment

          (1) Assess quantity and appearance of blood and nature of blood loss.

          (2) Assess degree of accompanying discomfort.

          (3) Assess family's coping mechanisms.

       e) Nursing diagnoses

          (1) Fear related to possible pregnancy loss

          (2) Pain related to abdominal cramping

          (3) Anticipatory grieving related to expected loss of fetus

       f) Nursing intervention

          (1) Provide reassurance and emotional support.

          (2) Explain why pain is occurring and provide analgesics as necessary.

       g) Nursing evaluation

          (1) Client understands nature of spontaneous abortion and knows possible impact on future pregnancies.

          (2) Client goes through appropriate grieving stages.

    2. Ectopic pregnancy (also known as tubal pregnancy): implantation of blastocyst in a site other than the uterine endometrial lining, usually in a fallopian tube

       a) Signs and symptoms

          (1) Initial: amenorrhea, breast tenderness, nausea, positive pregnancy test

          (2) Later (when fallopian tube ruptures and bleeding occurs into abdominal cavity): increased sharp pain, often referred to shoulder; vaginal bleeding; onset of shock

       b) Risk: maternal mortality

       c) Medical therapy

          (1) Diagnosis through menstrual history, physical exam, ultrasound, culdocentesis, laparotomy, laparoscopy

          (2) Surgical removal of products of conception from tube (salpingostomy); possible removal of fallopian tube (salpingectomy)

      (3) Monitoring for signs of shock and infection and treatment as appropriate

   d) Nursing assessment

      (1) Determine the appearance and amount of vaginal bleeding.

      (2) Monitor vital signs for development of hypovolemic shock.

      (3) Observe for signs of infection (e.g., pain, fever, elevated white blood count).

      (4) Observe client's and family's level of knowledge about condition and procedures and their coping abilities.

   e) Nursing diagnoses

      (1) Knowledge deficit related to ectopic pregnancy and its complications

      (2) Pain related to bleeding into abdominal cavity after rupture

      (3) Anticipatory grieving related to loss of fetus

   f) Nursing intervention

      (1) Teach client about the condition.

      (2) Provide analgesics.

      (3) Report signs of shock immediately.

      (4) Provide blood transfusions and IV fluids as needed.

      (5) Provide ongoing supportive care for client and family.

   g) Nursing evaluation

      (1) Client and family understand condition and procedures and how to be alert for postoperative complications (e.g., infection, hemorrhage, adhesion).

      (2) Client does not develop postoperative complications.

      (3) Client and family are able to express their grief.

      (4) Client and family understand chances for a future successful pregnancy.

3. Molar pregnancy (hydatidiform mole): gestational trophoblastic neoplasms that arise from chorionic villi

   a) Signs and symptoms

      (1) Early: cannot be distinguished from normal pregnancy

      (2) Later: vaginal bleeding, uterus larger than expected for date, anemia secondary to blood loss, excessive nausea and vomiting, abdominal cramping, possible PIH

   b) Risks: maternal development of choriocarcinoma, disseminated intravascular coagulation, iron deficiency anemia, lung embolization

   c) Medical therapy

      (1) Diagnosis confirmed by ultrasound

      (2) Dilatation and curettage

      (3) Follow-up care to detect malignancy

   d) Nursing assessment

      (1) Assess vital signs for elevated blood pressure.

      (2) Inspect vaginal blood, looking for clear, filled vesicles and dark-brown spotting.

      (3) Ascertain fundal height for height greater than normal for gestational age.

    (4) Assess for absence of fetal heart sounds and fetal activity.

    (5) Assess client's knowledge of condition and ability to cope.

   e) Nursing diagnoses

    (1) Anxiety related to diagnosis and potential malignancy

    (2) Altered nutrition related to nausea and vomiting

    (3) High risk for fluid volume deficit related to uterine bleeding

    (4) Grieving related to loss of pregnancy

   f) Nursing intervention

    (1) Teach client pathophysiology of molar pregnancy.

    (2) Advise client that hCG levels must be evaluated monthly for a year after removal of mole to identify any malignancy.

    (3) Advise a plan for contraception to prevent pregnancy for 1 year during follow-up testing (to prevent confusion about cause of elevated hCG levels).

    (4) Provide ongoing supportive care to client and family.

   g) Nursing evaluation

    (1) Client understands pathophysiology of condition.

    (2) Client accepts need to monitor hCG levels for early identification of malignancy.

    (3) Client accepts plan for contraception for 1 year.

  D. Bleeding (hemorrhagic) problems in late pregnancy

   1. Placenta previa: development of placenta in lower uterine segment so it partially or wholly covers cervix

    a) Contributing factors: previous history of placenta previa, multiparity, increasing maternal age, previous cesarean or other uterine surgery, multiple gestation

    b) Signs and symptoms (see Nurse Alert, "How to Distinguish Placenta Previa from Abruptio Placentae")

    c) Risks

     (1) Maternal: hypovolemic shock, hemorrhage, obstruction of birth canal

     (2) Fetal/neonatal: prematurity, hypoxia, intrauterine growth retardation, fetal malposition

    d) Medical therapy

     (1) Diagnosis through ultrasound

     (2) Diagnosis through double setup (if not diagnosable by ultrasound): pelvic exam performed in operating room in preparation for cesarean section, if placenta previa is confirmed and heavy bleeding occurs

     (3) Conservative management if bleeding is not excessive: bed rest and observation to allow fetus to mature

     (4) Delivery if client is in labor or if bleeding is excessive

How to Distinguish Placenta Previa from Abruptio Placentae

Placenta previa	Abruptio placentae
• Painless	• Severely painful
• Spotting or heavy bleeding	• Heavy bleeding, which may be partially or completely hidden
• Bright-red bleeding	• Usually dark-brown bleeding
• Soft, nontender, relaxed uterus with normal tone	• Rigid (possibly boardlike), tender uterus, possibly with contractions
• Shock in proportion to observed blood loss	• Shock seeming to be out of proportion to blood loss (if blood loss is concealed)
• Signs of fetal distress usually not present	• Signs of fetal distress

e) Nursing assessment
   (1) Assess vital signs and hemoglobin and hematocrit levels.
   (2) Assess amount of bleeding and color of blood.
   (3) Assess uterine activity: amount of pain and contractility.
   (4) Assess fetal heart rate pattern with electronic fetal monitor to detect possible onset of distress.
   (5) Assess family's coping mechanisms.
f) Nursing diagnoses
   (1) Potential for impaired fetal gas exchange related to blood loss
   (2) Risk for infection related to loss of cervical mucus plug
   (3) Fear related to loss of control over pregnancy outcome
   (4) Altered family processes related to need for prolonged bed rest and possible hospitalization
   (5) High risk for altered renal, cerebral, and peripheral tissue perfusion related to excessive blood loss
g) Nursing intervention
   (1) Teach client and family pathophysiology of disorder, including need for bed rest if condition is being managed conservatively.
   (2) Monitor blood loss, providing blood transfusions, IV fluids, and oxygen as needed.
   (3) Prepare client for possible cesarean delivery.
   (4) Provide ongoing supportive care to client and family.
h) Nursing evaluation
   (1) Client understands pathophysiology of condition.
   (2) Client observes need for bed rest.
   (3) Client maintains normal tissue perfusion, blood pressure, and pulse; urine output is >30 ml/hr; urine is clear and straw-colored.
   (4) Client and family are reassured about management of condition.
   (5) Client delivers healthy infant at or near term.

2. Abruptio placentae: premature separation of a normally located placenta from uterine attachment
    a) Types
        (1) Concealed, or internal: blood trapped behind uterine wall
        (2) Marginal, external: blood escapes through vagina
        (3) Complete: massive bleeding (>500 ml) internally and externally
    b) Contributing factors: maternal hypertension, grand multiparity (5 or more), trauma, maternal use of cocaine or alcohol, hydramnios, multiple gestation, smoking
    c) Signs and symptoms (see Nurse Alert, "How to Distinguish Placenta Previa from Abruptio Placentae")
    d) Risks
        (1) Maternal: hypovolemic shock, hemorrhage, disseminated intravascular coagulation, Couvelaire uterus, renal failure
        (2) Fetal/neonatal: prematurity, hypoxia, anoxia, neurologic damage, mortality
    e) Medical therapy
        (1) Diagnosis through ultrasound or CAT scan
        (2) Safe delivery of fetus (vaginal delivery if mild, cesarean if moderate to severe)
        (3) Control of hemorrhage
        (4) Laboratory tests to determine coagulation status
    f) Nursing assessment
        (1) Assess vital signs, hematocrit and hemoglobin levels, amount of bleeding, color of blood, and amount of pain.
        (2) Assess fetal heart rate with electronic fetal monitor to detect distress.
        (3) Determine changes in fundal height because increases are associated with concealed bleeding.
        (4) Monitor results of coagulation tests.
        (5) Assess family's coping mechanisms.
    g) Nursing diagnoses (same as section II,D,1,f of this chapter)
    h) Nursing intervention
        (1) Monitor blood loss, providing blood transfusions, IV fluids, and oxygen as needed.
        (2) Encourage client to lie in lateral recumbent position to increase venous return and blood available to placenta.
        (3) Prepare client for possible emergency cesarean section.
        (4) Provide ongoing supportive care to client and family.

i) Nursing evaluation
  (1) Client maintains normal tissue perfusion, blood pressure, and pulse; urine output is >30 ml/hour; urine is clear and straw-colored.
  (2) Client and family are reassured about management of condition.
  (3) Client delivers healthy infant.
  (4) In case of fetal/neonatal mortality, client and family are able to express grief appropriately.

E. Premature rupture of membranes (PROM): spontaneous rupture of amniotic membranes prior to onset of labor; may be preterm (before 38 weeks' gestation) or at term
  1. Contributing factors: incompetent os, infection, trauma
  2. Signs and symptoms: leakage of amniotic fluid; pH higher than 6.5, reactive to nitrazine paper
  3. Risks
    a) Maternal: infection (chorioamnionitis), endometritis, prolapsed cord
    b) Fetal/neonatal: infection, respiratory distress syndrome from preterm delivery, hypoxia
  4. Medical therapy: depends on gestational age and presence or absence of infection
    a) With infection: antibiotics and delivery of infant
    b) Without infection
      (1) Conservative treatment includes hospitalization for bed rest, monitoring of fetus and for infection; may be able to be home.
      (2) Betamethasone (glucocorticoid) may be given to accelerate fetal lung maturation and prevent respiratory distress syndrome.
  5. Nursing assessment
    a) Determine when rupture occurred to assess risk of infection and whether contractions have started.
    b) Monitor for signs of infection: review white blood cell count, temperature, pulse rate, and character (odor, color, amount) of amniotic fluid.
    c) Assess fetal heart rate pattern with electronic fetal monitor to detect possible onset of distress.
    d) Assess knowledge of client and family about condition and possible preterm cesarean delivery.
  6. Nursing diagnoses
    a) Knowledge deficit related to PROM, implications, and treatment
    b) High risk for infection related to loss of cervical mucus plug
    c) High risk for prolapsed cord related to loss of amniotic sac
    d) Ineffective individual and family coping related to possible need for hospitalization and restricted activity

7. Nursing intervention
   a) Record time of rupture and presence of contractions.
   b) Observe client for signs of infection.
   c) Teach client about PROM and treatment.
   d) Provide continuing supportive care to client and family.
8. Nursing evaluation
   a) Client understands her condition and the importance of restricted activity.
   b) Infection is prevented or controlled.
   c) Client delivers healthy infant at or near term.

F. Preterm labor: labor initiated between 20 and 37 weeks
   1. Contributing factors: PROM, history of multiple abortions, abdominal surgery while pregnant, infection, placenta previa, pregnancy-induced hypertension (PIH), hydramnios, multiple gestation
   2. Signs and symptoms (see Client Teaching Checklist, "Home Monitoring Program for Preterm Labor")
   3. Risks
      a) Maternal: anxiety over delivering nonviable or high-risk preterm fetus and possible prolonged bed rest
      b) Fetal/neonatal: breech presentation, respiratory distress syndrome, prematurity, mortality
   4. Medical therapy
      a) Early detection of preterm labor
      b) Suppression of advancing labor through bed rest and drug therapy
      c) Tocolytic drugs: used to suppress preterm labor, usually by inhibiting uterine contractions
         (1) Beta-adrenergic agonists: ritodrine (Yutopar), terbutaline (Brethine); intravenous administration initially, then oral long-term maintenance if contractions stop, *or* delivery of medication with subcutaneous infusion pump
         (2) Magnesium sulfate ($MgSO_4$): used when ritodrine or terbutaline is ineffective or when side effects contraindicate the use of these drugs
   5. Nursing assessment
      a) Assess vital signs, contraction pattern, and presence of contributing factors for preterm labor.
      b) Assess fetal heart rate pattern with electronic fetal monitor to detect possible onset of distress.
      c) Assess progress of preterm labor, effects of treatment, and physiologic impact on client and fetus.

Home Monitoring Program for Preterm Labor

Tell client to report these signs to a health care provider:

✔ Uterine contractions that occur every 10 minutes or less for 1 hour (uterine activity to be evaluated once or twice a day)
✔ Menstrual-like cramps felt low in the abdomen for 1 hour
✔ Constant or recurring pelvic pressure for 1 hour
✔ Constant or recurring dull ache in lower back for 1 hour
✔ Abdominal cramping, possibly accompanied by diarrhea, for 1 hour
✔ Increased bloody show or clear fluid leaking from vagina

6. Nursing diagnoses
   a) Knowledge deficit related to causes, identification, and treatment of preterm labor
   b) Anticipatory grieving related to risk for preterm birth
   c) Ineffective individual and family coping related to loss of control regarding pregnancy outcome
7. Nursing intervention
   a) Identify high-risk client.
   b) Teach client and family about signs and symptoms, how to evaluate fetal activity 1–2 times per day, and how to use home monitoring system to evaluate uterine changes.
   c) Promote bed rest, placing client on side; monitor vital signs, fetal heart rate pattern, and uterine contractions.
   d) Monitor for evidence of side effects from tocolytic agents, MgSO$_4$ toxicity (see Nurse Alerts, "Observing for Side Effects of Beta-Adrenergic Agonists" and "Observing for Signs of MgSO$_4$ Toxicity").
   e) Provide ongoing supportive care to client and family.
8. Nursing evaluation
   a) Client understands condition and how to evaluate fetal activity, contractions, and potential tocolytic side effects.
   b) Client is compliant with restricted activity.
   c) Client and family are reassured about management of condition.
   d) Client delivers healthy infant at or near term.

III. Maternal psychosocial and behavioral risk factors

See text pages
_____

A. Poverty
   1. Low-income clients tend to become pregnant at early age, have more pregnancies, and less time between pregnancies, causing increase in perinatal risks to client and fetus.
   2. Risks include preterm delivery and low-birth-weight infants, intercurrent illness, and obstetric complications (hemorrhage and placental insufficiency).

3. Essential nursing care involves assisting client in locating resources to meet her needs for financial aid and health care.

B. Spousal abuse
   1. Women at all socioeconomic and educational levels are affected.
   2. Pregnancy increases the likelihood of domestic violence.
   3. Risks include preterm labor, abruptio placentae, low-birth-weight infant, and fetal mortality.

! NURSE *ALERT* !

Observing for Side Effects of Beta-Adrenergic Agonists

Monitor for these maternal side effects:
- Pulmonary edema (be alert to decreased breath sounds and client complaints of difficulty catching breath)
- Tachycardia (notify physician if >120 beats/minute)
- Increased systolic blood pressure and decreased diastolic blood pressure
- Premature ventricular contractions (PVCs)
- Hyperglycemia
- Hypokalemia
- Palpitations
- Tremors
- Nausea and vomiting
- Headache
- Muscle weakness
- Dyspnea
- Nervousness
- Chest pain
- Cardiac arrhythmias

Monitor for these fetal-neonatal side effects:
- Tachycardia (notify physician if >180 beats/minute)
- Hypoglycemia
- PVCs
- Acidosis
- Hypoxia

Treatment:
- Discontinue therapy if pulmonary edema or cardiac problems occur.
- Beta-blocking agents should be available as antidote.

4. Essential nursing care includes identifying battered client, allowing client to express fears, helping client investigate her options, finding community resources to help her.

C. Teratogens: substances that cause harm to fetus (most detrimental effect during first trimester when fetal organs are being formed)
   1. Psychoactive drugs
      a) Alcohol abuse
         (1) Maternal risks: poor nutrition, inadequate or nonexistent prenatal care, possible withdrawal seizures within 12–48 hours after alcohol cessation
         (2) Fetal risks: fetal alcohol syndrome (FAS)
            (a) Growth deficit at birth that does not improve with time
            (b) Neurologic dysfunction since brain is most sensitive to damage from alcohol
            (c) Possible feeding difficulties
            (d) Facial dysmorphology
      b) Illicit drug abuse (cocaine, heroin, methamphetamine)
         (1) Maternal risks: general health deterioration; increased risk of infection; poor nutritional level; high risk of STD, PIH, preterm labor, abruptio placentae, AIDS
         (2) Fetal/neonatal risks: intrauterine asphyxia as a result of fetal withdrawal secondary to maternal withdrawal; severe decrease in uteroplacental blood flow; placental insufficiency; low birth weight with low Apgar scores, respiratory distress syndrome, jaundice, congenital anomalies, and growth retardation; learning disabilities
   2. Cigarette smoking: linked to increased risk of spontaneous abortion, placental abruption, preterm labor, low birth weight, and intrauterine growth retardation
   3. Prescription and over-the-counter medications
      a) Teratogenic effects are not clear in all cases; all medications should be avoided, if possible.
      b) Food and Drug Administration (FDA) has categories of medications given during pregnancy: A, B, C, D, X (from no known risk to risk that clearly outweighs value of drug).
      c) Drugs in high-risk categories (D and X) include tetracycline, lithium, and estrogens.
   4. Environmental and occupational hazards
      a) Inhaled substances are the most common concern.
      b) Types include pesticides, lead, glycol esters, vinyl chloride (aerosol spray), antineoplastic agents, polychlorinated biphenyl (PCB), radiation (x-rays), video display terminals, and anesthetics.
      c) Risk depends on exposure level, dose, and length of time.
      d) Some individuals are more susceptible than others.
      e) Risks include miscarriage, growth retardation, chromosomal aberrations, and prematurity.

5. Infection (see section I,F of this chapter)
6. Essential nursing care includes assessment of use of or exposure to teratogenic substances by client, client teaching about harmful effect of teratogens, referral to drug or alcohol counseling services as appropriate, drug screen for high-risk clients on admission to labor and delivery, and notification of nursery personnel of possible drug use.

See text pages
_____

IV. Tests to screen and diagnose fetal well-being

A. Ultrasound: based on returning echo of directional beam of sound striking an object; can visualize fetus in utero
  1. Types: transabdominal and endovaginal
  2. Purposes
    a) First trimester: to look for gestational sac, fetal cardiac and body movements, and uterine abnormalities; pregnancy dating using 2 measurements
      (1) Biparietal diameter of fetal head
      (2) Crown-to-rump length of fetus
    b) Second and third trimesters: to look for fetal growth (intrauterine growth retardation [IUGR], small for gestational age [SGA], large for gestational age [LGA]), anatomy, fetal heart rate, and volume of amniotic fluid; to assess for placental, uterine, or congenital abnormalities
  3. Advantages: noninvasive, painless, provides serial assessment for comparison, gives immediate results, is safe (no ionizing radiation), can differentiate soft tissue masses
  4. Disadvantages: decreased accuracy of findings for fetal gestation if no baseline sonogram was obtained in early pregnancy

B. Biophysical monitoring: tests during third trimester for evaluating fetus in high-risk pregnancy
  1. Nonstress test (NST)
    a) Purpose: to observe acceleration of fetal heart rate with fetal movement
    b) Results
      (1) Reactive pattern (2 or more accelerations of 15 beats/minute lasting 15 seconds) suggests fetal well-being.
      (2) Nonreactive pattern (no accelerations or accelerations of less than 15 beats/minute or lasting less than 15 seconds) requires further testing.

    c) Advantages: does not require intravenous drugs, is inexpensive, can be done on outpatient basis, has no known side effects

    d) Disadvantages: may not give proper tracing and requires client to remain still for an extended time

2. Contraction stress test (CST): observation of fetal heart rate in presence of induced or spontaneous contractions

    a) Types

        (1) Oxytocin-induced contractions

        (2) Nipple-stimulated contractions

    b) Purpose: to evaluate respiratory function (oxygen and carbon dioxide exchange) of the placenta

    c) Results (based on theory that healthy fetus can normally withstand a decreased oxygen supply during physiologic stress of contraction)

        (1) No late decelerations and minimum of 3 contractions in 10 minutes indicate negative, or normal, outcome.

        (2) Occurrence of repeated late decelerations with contractions is positive, or abnormal, test.

    d) Advantages

        (1) Both types: can be done on an outpatient basis

        (2) Nipple stimulation test: is noninvasive and costs less and takes less time than oxytocin test

    e) Disadvantages

        (1) Both types: must be done in or near labor/birth unit because of possibility of labor onset, fetal heart rate decelerations, uterine tetany

        (2) Oxytocin test: requires IV medication and is lengthy procedure (90 minutes)

        (3) Nipple stimulation test: embarrassment of client

3. Fetal biophysical profile: fetal surveillance based on a composite assessment of several markers of fetal distress

    a) Purpose: to identify compromised fetus

    b) Variables used in assessment

        (1) Fetal breathing movements, gross body movements, fetal tone, qualitative amniotic fluid volume (assessed with ultrasound)

        (2) Reactive fetal heart rate (assessed with nonstress test)

    c) Results

        (1) Score of 2 is given for each normal assessment finding.

        (2) Score of 0 is given for each abnormal finding.

        (3) Total score of 8–10 indicates overall normal fetus with low risk of chronic asphyxia, unless decreased amniotic fluid is found.

C. Maternal assessment (see Client Teaching Checklist, "Methods of Assessment of Fetal Activity by Pregnant Woman," in Chapter 5)

D. Alpha-fetoprotein (AFP) screening: analysis of maternal blood for presence and volume of AFP; done between 15 and 18 weeks of gestation
   1. Results
      a) Elevated levels are associated with neural tube defects such as spina bifida and anencephaly. (If levels are elevated, test should be repeated 1–2 weeks after initial test.)
      b) Decreased levels are predictive of some congenital abnormalities (trisomies).
   2. Must be followed up with ultrasound, amniocentesis, or chromosomal analysis

E. Amniocentesis: analysis of amniotic fluid
   1. Purposes
      a) To identify genetic problems by karyotyping fluid for chromosomal abnormalities
      b) To detect sex and inborn errors of metabolism
      c) To obtain amniotic AFP for neural tube defect testing
      d) To ascertain fetal maturity by level of lung development
      e) To assess fetal hemolytic disease, indicated by increased concentration in amniotic fluid of bilirubin and other red blood cell breakdown products
   2. Procedure
      a) Fluid withdrawn by transabdominal aspiration
      b) Performed after 14th week when sufficient amniotic fluid is available
      c) Ultrasound performed first to determine location of fetus, placenta, and pockets of amniotic fluid as well as during testing
   3. Risks: less than 1% for pregnant woman and fetus
      a) Maternal: hemorrhage; infection; initiation of labor; amniotic fluid embolism; trauma to placenta, umbilical cord, or maternal structures
      b) Fetal: death, hemorrhage, infection, injury from needle, abortion, preterm labor, trauma

F. Chorionic villus sampling (CVS): alternative to amniocentesis
   1. Provides earlier diagnosis of fetal genetic disorders, gives faster results, allows first trimester therapeutic abortion
   2. Procedure: transcervical aspiration of chorionic tissue from placental site
   3. Risks
      a) Maternal: infection and spontaneous abortion
      b) Fetal: congenital anomalies, intrauterine growth retardation, Rh isoimmunization

4. May require follow-up with amniocentesis or percutaneous umbilical blood sampling (PUBS)

G. Essential nursing care
1. Explain procedure.
2. Answer client's questions and discuss concerns.
3. Prepare client for testing (e.g., attach IV and attach electronic fetal monitor) as appropriate.
4. Monitor client and fetus during and after procedure.
5. Document results.
6. Assist in interpreting and explaining results to client.
7. Refer client for genetic counseling if needed.

1. During a routine prenatal visit, Tonya, 36 weeks pregnant, states that she has difficulty breathing and a rapid pulse. She tells the nurse that she is always very tired and her shoes are now too tight. The nurse finds Tonya's pulse to be 100 and irregular with bilateral crackles in lower lung bases. The best nursing diagnosis based on these data is:

   a. Altered tissue perfusion related to hypotensive syndrome.

   b. Ineffective gas exchange related to pulmonary congestion.

   c. Activity intolerance related to increased metabolic requirements of pregnancy.

   d. Anxiety related to fear of pregnancy outcomes.

2. Tonya is hospitalized and placed on complete bed rest. She asks the nurse, "Can I have visitors?" The best response for the nurse is:

   a. "No, you need absolute quiet and no extra stimulation."

   b. "Are you really up for it?"

   c. "Yes, but be sure that no one has a cold or the flu."

   d. "Only if you agree to stay in bed while they are here."

3. Heidi, age 25, has type I diabetes. She is 10 weeks pregnant and has had persistent nausea and vomiting. She states that her blood glucose has been 60–80 mg/dl. The nurse is concerned that Heidi is at risk to develop:

   a. Hypoglycemia.

   b. Hyperglycemia.

   c. Ketoacidosis.

   d. Glycosuria.

4. Heidi has a glycosylated hemoglobin (A_1) of 12%. At this time, the nurse should be most concerned about which of the following possible fetal outcomes?

   a. Incompetent cervix

   b. Abruptio placentae

   c. Placenta previa

   d. Spontaneous abortion

5. When Heidi is at 32 weeks' gestation, she has a reactive nonstress test (NST). This finding suggests:

   a. Fetal well-being.

   b. That further testing is needed.

   c. That an emergency cesarean section is needed.

   d. Fetal demise.

6. Jolanda is HIV-positive and at 32 weeks' gestation. She tells the nurse that she would like to breastfeed her infant. The nurse should:

   a. Encourage breastfeeding to facilitate bonding.

   b. Encourage breastfeeding because of breast milk's antibacterial and antiviral properties.

   c. Discourage breastfeeding since HIV can be transmitted in breast milk.

   d. Discourage breastfeeding because Jolanda will need to rest.

7. A client is admitted to the hospital with preeclampsia. Her blood pressure is 148/100, her proteinuria is 2+, and she has pitting ankle edema. She is started on magnesium sulfate ($MgSO_4$) intravenously. The nurse should have available at the bedside:

   a. Naloxone (Narcon).

   b. Calcium gluconate.

   c. Epinephrine.

   d. Diazepam (Valium).

8. Amanda, at 32 weeks' gestation, is admitted from the emergency room to the labor and delivery unit with a diagnosis of abruptio placentae. The nurse could expect Amanda to have:

   a. Bright-red bleeding.
   b. Soft, nontender uterus.
   c. Elevated temperature.
   d. Severe, sharp abdominal pain.

9. The best position for Amanda is:

   a. Left lateral recumbent.
   b. Supine.
   c. High-Fowler's.
   d. Trendelenburg's.

10. Rita, at 28 weeks' gestation, is receiving home care for preterm labor. She also receives oral ritodrine. During a visit from the nurse, Rita asks if she and her husband can have any sexual activity. The nurse's best response is that the couple may engage in:

    a. Cuddling and kissing.
    b. Nipple and breast stimulation.
    c. Intercourse using side-lying position.
    d. Mutual masturbation.

11. Katie, age 16, has been prescribed 300 mg of ferrous sulfate daily for her pregnancy-related anemia. To evaluate compliance, the nurse should:

    a. Assess hemoglobin and hematocrit level.
    b. Do a guaiac stool test.
    c. Weigh Katie.
    d. Ask Katie if she is taking the medication.

12. The most appropriate diet for a woman with preeclampsia is:

    a. High-protein, low-fiber, low-fat.
    b. High-protein, high-calorie, salt-restricted.
    c. Low-protein, low-fat, low-salt.
    d. High-protein, high-calorie, no added salt.

ANSWERS

1. **Correct answer is b.** The data presented (i.e., fatigue, dyspnea, rapid pulse, edema, and crackles) are classic signs of pulmonary edema and cardiac decompensation.

   a. Data presented do not support the etiology of hypotensive syndrome.
   c. Only fatigue indicates activity intolerance.
   d. Data presented do not support diagnosis of anxiety.

2. **Correct answer is c.** Tonya could have visitors, but no one with upper respiratory infections should be allowed. Should Tonya contract an infection, further demands would be placed on her heart.

   a. Tonya does not need absolute quiet.
   b. This statement does not answer Tonya's question.
   d. Tonya is already on bed rest regardless of whether or not she has visitors.

3. **Correct answer is a.** Heidi is at risk for hypoglycemia since her nausea and vomiting may prevent absorption of adequate caloric intake. Because there is a significant transfer of glucose to the embryo and fetus during the first trimester, Heidi is more at risk for hypoglycemia than for other conditions listed.

   b and **c.** During the second trimester, Heidi would be at risk for developing hyperglycemia since increasing insulin antagonist factors are present that will require greater amounts of insulin for Heidi. Uncorrected hyperglycemia can lead to diabetic ketoacidosis.
   d. Glycosuria occurs during the normal course of pregnancy due to lowered renal threshold to glucose excretion.

4. **Correct answer is d.** Glycosylated hemoglobin in the person with diabetes is an indicator of average serum glucose over the previous 4–12 weeks. Normal range is 6%–8%. The degree of increase relates inversely to the degree of long-term plasma glucose concentration. Studies indicate high levels are associated with spontaneous abortions as well as congenital abnormalities. Additionally, spontaneous abortion normally occurs early in pregnancy.

   a. An incompetent cervix or dilatation of the cervical os without labor or contractions may result in a miscarriage or preterm delivery. However, it is not related to glycosylated hemoglobin.
   b. Abruptio placentae occurs after the 20th week.
   c. Placenta previa occurs most often in the second trimester.

5. **Correct answer is a.** A nonstress test that is reactive suggests fetal well-being. It indicates that there was acceleration of fetal heart rate with fetal movement.

   b. Had the results of the nonstress test been nonreactive, Heidi would require further testing, most likely a contraction stress test (CST).
   c and d. These situations are not indicated with a reactive pattern.

6. **Correct answer is c.** Transmission of HIV to the infant can occur through breast milk.

   a. Even though breastfeeding does facilitate bonding, a mother who is HIV-positive should not do it.
   b. The chance of transmitting HIV through breast milk overrides its antibacterial and antiviral properties.
   d. Breastfeeding should be discouraged but for the reason given in correct answer c.

7. **Correct answer is b.** Calcium gluconate is used to antagonize the effects of $MgSO_4$ and should be readily available when a client is receiving $MgSO_4$.

   a. Naloxone is used as the antidote for narcotic toxicity.
   c. Epinephrine is a beta-adrenergic agonist used as a bronchodilator and cardiac stimulant.
   d. Diazepam is used as an anticonvulsant.

8. **Correct answer is d.** A characteristic sign of abruptio placentae is sharp, "knifelike" abdominal pain. This may or may not be accompanied by heavy, visible bleeding.

   a and b. These are characteristics of placenta previa.
   c. An elevated temperature is seen in inflammatory and infectious processes.

9. **Correct answer is a.** The left lateral recumbent position is used to facilitate maternal venous blood return and to increase perfusion to the placenta.

   b. The supine position would not be used since uterine/fetal weight would decrease flow of blood through the maternal vena cava.
   c. The high-Fowler's position would not facilitate placental perfusion.
   d. The Trendelenburg's position may be used when clients are in shock.

10. **Correct answer is a.** Rita would want to avoid activities that could stimulate labor. Affection received through hugs, cuddling, and kissing would be appropriate.

    b. Nipple stimulation may cause release of oxytocin, which can increase uterine activity.
    c. Intercourse is prohibited since prostaglandins in semen can stimulate labor.
    d. Masturbation leading to orgasm should be discouraged because it can cause uterine stimulation and contractions.

11. **Correct answer is a.** When the client is taking iron supplements, the nurse should see an increase in hemoglobin level over time.

    b. A guaiac stool test, which determines presence of blood in stool, is not evaluative of iron supplementation.

    c. Weight may reflect nutritional intake. However, it is not specific for iron intake.

    d. The client may or may not respond truthfully to the question.

12. **Correct answer is d.** A preeclamptic woman needs increased protein since she is losing protein through the urine. She also needs high calories to meet fetal and maternal nutritional needs in a stressful condition. She does not need to restrict salt intake but should not add it to her diet.

    a. High protein is appropriate. However, all pregnant women need to have an adequate amount of fiber to prevent constipation, and a normal intake of fat is allowed.

    b. There is no need to restrict salt intake. In fact, doing so may lead to other problems.

    c. A preeclamptic client, for the reason stated in correct answer d, needs increased protein. Low fat and low salt are not required.

7

Labor and Delivery (Childbirth)

1. The birth process includes factors related to the size of the fetus, the shape and size of the maternal pelvis, the forces acting to expel the fetus, and maternal psychologic preparation for labor and delivery.
2. Intrapartal assessment includes attention to the physical and psychologic needs of the mother as well as ongoing monitoring of the fetus.
3. Pain during delivery is affected by both physical factors and the maternal response to the pain.
4. Various methods and medications are available to control pain, and the choice is made based on maternal preference and the clinical circumstances.
5. Nurse must be nonjudgmental and supportive regarding clients' responses to pain.
6. An important part of nursing care is to give quiet reassurance throughout the labor process, which is a time of crisis.
7. Priorities of nursing care are established based on the assessment of physiologic and psychologic factors.
8. Behavioral responses to labor vary with the phase of labor and the woman's preparation, previous experience, cultural beliefs, developmental level, and support system.
9. A critical component of the birthing process is allowing the parents time and privacy for initiating attachment to their new baby.

GLOSSARY

episiotomy—surgical incision of maternal vulvar orifice to protect perineum, sphincter, and rectum from lacerations during childbirth; usually performed with regional or local anesthesia; repair occurs after birth and before or after placental expulsion

fetoscope—special stethoscope used for listening to fetal heart rate

fundus—upper portion of uterus between fallopian tubes

ischial spines—bony projections into midpelvis from ischial bones; used as reference points in determining fetal station

myometrium—layer of muscle in uterine wall

tocotransducer—external electronic monitoring instrument that records frequency and duration of contractions by means of pressure-sensing device

ultrasonic transducer—external electronic device that monitors fetal heart rate through use of high-frequency sound waves

ENHANCED OUTLINE

I. Essentials in labor

See text pages
_____

A. Passageway: pelvis
  1. Divisions of pelvis: true pelvis and false pelvis
     a) False pelvis is above the pelvic inlet, or brim; it supports pregnant uterus and directs fetus into true pelvis.
     b) True pelvis is divided into three parts: the inlet; the midpelvis, or pelvic cavity; and the outlet. Size and shape must be adequate for vaginal delivery.
  2. Pelvic measurements
     a) Pelvic inlet
        (1) Anteroposterior diameters
           (a) Diagonal conjugate
              i) Extends from lower border of symphysis pubis to sacral promontory
              ii) Can be measured manually through vaginal examination (should be at least 11.5 cm)
           (b) True conjugate, or conjugata vera
           (c) Obstetric conjugate (most significant measurement)
              i) Length usually estimated by subtracting 1.5–2 cm from diagonal conjugate measurement
              ii) Determines whether presenting part of fetus can engage, or enter, inlet
        (2) Transverse diameter: largest diameter of inlet (13 cm or more); greatest diameter of fetal head accommodates itself to this diameter as it enters inlet
     b) Midpelvis
        (1) Adequacy of midpelvis for vaginal delivery is measured by determining prominence of ischial spines.
        (2) Midpelvis contains the smallest part of the pelvis (plane of least dimensions).
     c) Pelvic outlet
        (1) Anteroposterior diameter: 11.5 cm
        (2) Transverse diameter (also called intertuberous or bi-ischial diameter): 8 cm or more; largest diameter of fetal head accommodates itself to this outlet diameter
        (3) Posterior sagittal diameter: 9 cm
  3. Pelvic types
     a) Gynecoid: round; all diameters adequate for vaginal delivery
     b) Android: heart-shaped, "male" pelvis; inadequate for vaginal delivery

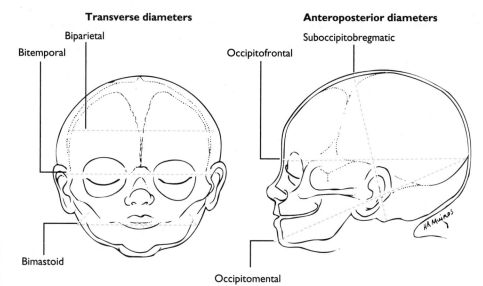

Transverse diameters

Bitemporal

Biparietal

Bimastoid

Anteroposterior diameters

Suboccipitobregmatic

Occipitofrontal

Occipitomental

Figure 7-1
Fetal Head Measurements

    c) Anthropoid: oval, narrow side to side and widened front to back; adequate for vaginal delivery

    d) Platypelloid: flat; usually inadequate for vaginal delivery

B. Passenger: fetus

  1. Fetal skull is composed of 2 frontal bones, 2 parietal bones, and 1 occipital bone.

    a) Bones are not knit together.

    b) Bones are separated by membranous interspaces called sutures; points at which sutures intersect are called fontanels.

      (1) Sutures: sagittal, lambdoidal, coronal, frontal

      (2) Fontanels: anterior (diamond-shaped), posterior (triangular)

    c) Sutures allow bones to overlap during labor, reducing fetal head size (molding).

    d) After rupture of membranes during labor, palpation of sutures and fontanels during vaginal exam helps determine fetal presentation, position, and attitude.

    e) If head can pass safely, the rest of the body can usually be delivered without difficulty.

    f) Significant fetal head measurements are listed.

      (1) Biparietal diameter: largest transverse diameter (9.5–9.8 cm); represents the greatest width of fetal head

      (2) Suboccipitobregmatic diameter: smallest anteroposterior diameter (9.5 cm); occurs when fetal head is totally flexed

      (3) Occipitomental diameter: largest anteroposterior diameter (13.5 cm); occurs when fetal head is markedly extended

2. Fetal lie is the relationship of the long (cephalocaudal) axis, or spine, of the fetus to the same axis of the woman.
   a) Longitudinal lie: Long axis of fetus is parallel to woman's long axis (99% of labors at term).
   b) Transverse lie: Long axis of fetus is at right angle to woman's long axis (1% of labors at term).
3. Fetal presentation is that part of the fetus that enters the pelvis first and is determined by fetal lie.
   a) Cephalic (head): most common; further defined by position of fetal head
      (1) Vertex: head flexed with chin on chest
      (2) Face: head completely extended with occiput on fetal back
      (3) Brow: head partially extended

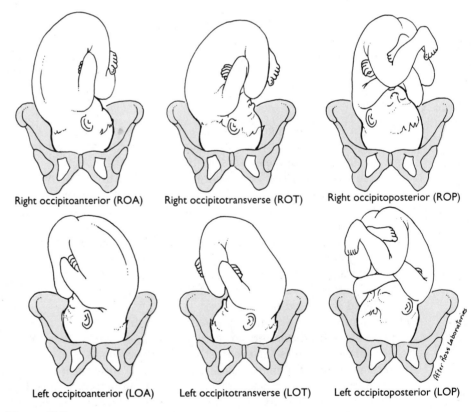

Right occipitoanterior (ROA) Right occipitotransverse (ROT) Right occipitoposterior (ROP)

Left occipitoanterior (LOA) Left occipitotransverse (LOT) Left occipitoposterior (LOP)

After Ross Laboratories

Figure 7-2
Fetal Presentations: Vertex

Face presentations

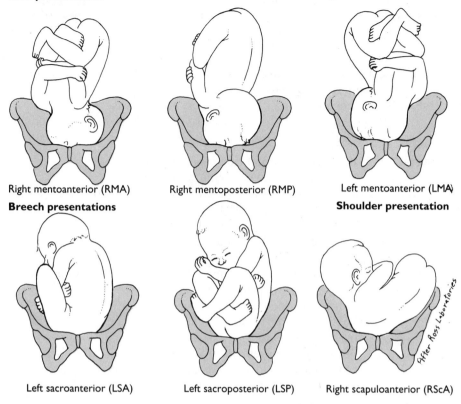

Right mentoanterior (RMA)   Right mentoposterior (RMP)   Left mentoanterior (LMA)

Breech presentations   **Shoulder presentation**

Left sacroanterior (LSA)   Left sacroposterior (LSP)   Right scapuloanterior (RScA)

After Ross Laboratories

Figure 7-3
Fetal Presentations: Face, Breech, Shoulder

      b) Breech (buttocks or lower extremities): frank, complete, or incomplete (footling) (see Chapter 8 Glossary for breech definitions)

      c) Shoulder (scapula): transverse lie with fetal spine perpendicular to maternal spine

4. Fetal attitude is the relationship of fetal parts to one another.

      a) Normal attitude: moderate flexion of head, flexion of arms and legs

      b) Deviations: larger diameters of fetal head presented to maternal pelvis, contributing to difficult labor

5. Fetal position is the relationship of the position of the presenting part (landmark) to the maternal pelvis.

      a) Position is identified by 3 letters: *R* or *L* to designate whether the fetal landmark is directed toward the right or left side of maternal pelvis; *O, M, S,* or *Sc* to designate a particular landmark on fetal presenting part (*O* is occiput [back of head], *M* is mentum [face], *S* is sacrum [bottom of spine], *Sc* is scapula [shoulder]); and *A, P,* or *T* to designate whether fetal landmark is directed toward anterior, posterior, or transverse position of maternal pelvis.

b) Station is the relationship of presenting part to imaginary line between maternal ischial spines.
  (1) Determines the rate of descent of the fetus
  (2) Is expressed in terms of centimeters above or below ischial spines

C. Powers: the forces acting to expel the fetus and placenta
  1. Primary powers: involuntary uterine contractions
    a) Divided into three phases: increment (building up), acme (peak), and decrement (letting down)
    b) Described in terms of:
      (1) Frequency: time between beginning of one contraction and beginning of next contraction
      (2) Duration: beginning of increment to completion of decrement
      (3) Intensity: strength of contraction during acme
    c) Effects of contractions in first stage of labor
      (1) Effacement: shortening and thinning of the cervix during the first stage of labor
      (2) Dilatation: enlargement or widening of cervical os and cervical canal to allow descent of presenting part into vagina (Ferguson's reflex: mechanical stretching of cervix intensifies uterine activity)
    d) Uterine anatomy
      (1) Upper segment of the corpus (known as the fundus): the active, contractile portion
      (2) Middle segment, or isthmus: passive portion (known in pregnancy as lower uterine segment)
      (3) Lowest segment, or cervix: composed of external and internal os
  2. Secondary powers: voluntary bearing-down effort using abdominal muscles
    a) Occurs in second stage of labor, when cervix is fully dilated and presenting part reaches pelvic floor
    b) Results in expulsion of fetus
    c) Has no effect on dilatation of cervix and is counterproductive when tried before cervix is fully dilated

D. Psyche
  1. Client's preparation for labor may include a variety of psychologic activities.
  2. Client can prepare through imaginary rehearsal, including use of breathing activities, distraction, simulated pushing exercises.
  3. Client can anticipate the labor in fantasy, including expressing her fear of pain.

4. Client's support system can influence course of labor and birth.
5. Client must deal with possible loss of control of bodily functions and changing emotions.

II. Premonitory signs of labor

See text pages
_____

A. Lightening: descent of fetal head into pelvis; accompanied by possible leg pain due to pressure on sciatic nerve, vaginal changes, and increased urinary frequency
   1. For primigravidas, usually occurs in last month of pregnancy
   2. For multigravidas, usually occurs immediately before or in labor

B. Braxton Hicks contractions: intermittent, usually painless contractions of uterus that are often mistaken for true labor

C. False labor: exaggerated Braxton Hicks contractions, often with discomfort, that occur close to term (see Nurse Alert, "Distinguishing False Labor from True Labor")

D. Vaginal show: mucus from mucous plug in cervical os mixed with blood from ruptured cervical capillaries

E. Rupture of membranes: leading to spontaneous labor within 24 hours in 80% of women (see Chapter 6, section II,E, for information on premature rupture of membranes)
   1. Danger of prolapsed umbilical cord if presenting part does not cover cervix (see Chapter 8, sections I,B,4,e–h, for nursing care of prolapsed cord)
   2. Client at increased risk for infection

F. Cervical changes: softening (ripening) of cervix and beginning of effacement and dilatation

G. General maternal response: possible loss of 1–3 lb of fluid weight and burst of energy ("nesting instinct")

❗ NURSE *ALERT* ❗

Distinguishing False Labor from True Labor

	False	True
• Contractions	Irregular intervals	Regular intervals
• Intervals	No change	Gradually shorten
• Duration	No change	Gradually increases
• Discomfort	In abdomen	In back, radiating around to abdomen
• Intensity	Lessened or not affected by walking	Gradually increases; walking increases intensity
• Cervical changes	No change	Progressive dilatation and effacement

See text pages

_____

III. Stages of labor

A. First (dilating) stage: begins with onset of true labor and ends when cervix completely dilated (10 cm); divided into 3 phases
   1. Latent phase: Uterine contractions become established and increase in frequency, intensity, and duration; cervix dilates from 0 to 3–4 cm.
      a) Duration: 8.6 hours (nullipara), 5.3 hours (multipara)
      b) Contractions: every 15–30 minutes, lasting 15–30 seconds
      c) Maternal response: usually able to cope with discomfort; anxious yet excited
   2. Active phase: Cervix dilates from 3–4 cm to 8 cm; fetal descent is progressive.
      a) Duration: 4.6 hours (nullipara), 2.4 hours (multipara)
      b) Contractions: every 3–5 minutes, lasting up to 60 seconds
      c) Maternal response: may be increasingly anxious and uncomfortable, nauseated, may vomit
   3. Transition phase: Cervical dilatation reaches 8–10 cm; fetal descent progresses; rupture of membranes may occur.
      a) Duration: 3 hours (nullipara), 1 hour (multipara)
      b) Contractions: every 2–3 minutes, lasting 60–90 seconds
      c) Maternal response: increasingly anxious, possible fear of abandonment, inner directed, pain most acute

B. Second (pushing) stage: begins when cervix completely dilated (10 cm) and ends with birth of baby
   1. Combination of forces helps move fetus.
      a) Uterine contractions become stronger, longer, and more frequent.
      b) Client experiences urge to bear down and use abdominal muscles, increasing intra-abdominal pressure.
   2. Rupture of membranes usually occurs, if it has not happened earlier.
   3. Perineum begins to bulge, flatten, and move anteriorly.
   4. Fetal head is gradually encircled by the external opening of vagina, called crowning; birth is imminent.
   5. Some clients may feel relieved that acute pain of transition phase is over and pushing can begin; others may feel fear and loss of control.
   6. Second stage lasts approximately 30–90 minutes (nullipara), 10–60 minutes (multipara).

C. Third (placental) stage: begins with birth of baby and ends with expulsion of placenta
   1. Placental separation: usually occurs within 5 minutes of delivery
      a) Uterus becomes globular and firmer and rises into abdomen.
      b) Umbilical cord descends 3 inches or more out of vagina.
      c) Sudden gush of blood occurs.

2. Placental expulsion: Client bears down on uterine fundus.
   a) Types of expulsion
      (1) Schultze mechanism: shiny presentation of fetal side of placenta
      (2) Duncan mechanism: dark, roughened presentation of maternal side of placenta
   b) Retained placenta: placenta not expelled within 30 minutes after completion of second stage of labor
3. Contractions: Uterus continues contracting, promoting hemostasis.
4. Maternal response: eager to explore baby, elated, fatigued
5. Duration: 5–30 minutes

D. Fourth (physiologic and psychologic readjustment) stage
   1. Restoration of physiologic stability
      a) Redistribution of blood into venous beds
      b) Myometrial contraction and retraction to control bleeding at placental site
      c) Restoration of firmness to fundus
   2. Bonding: important time for consolidation of family unit
   3. Duration: 1–4 hours

IV. Physiologic response of client and fetus to labor

See text pages
_____

A. Maternal response to labor
   1. Cardiovascular: Cardiac output and blood pressure increase; pulse slows.
   2. Respiratory
      a) Rate of respiration and oxygen consumption increase.
      b) The pH may increase early in labor (due to hyperventilation) but returns to normal by end of first stage.
   3. Fluid and electrolyte balance
      a) Perspiration and insensible water increase.
      b) Temperature may rise.
   4. Gastrointestinal
      a) Gastric motility and absorption of food decrease.
      b) Nausea may occur as reflex response to full dilatation of cervix.
   5. Renal: Bladder is pushed forward and upward.
      a) Interferes with ability to void spontaneously
      b) May exacerbate tissue edema
   6. Hematopoietic
      a) Leukocyte levels may increase to 25,000/mm³ as a stress response.
      b) Clotting factors increase during pregnancy and labor; after delivery of placenta, they decrease; they protect against hemorrhage during birth but place client at risk for thrombophlebitis after delivery.

B. Fetal response to labor
   1. Fetal position changes
      a) Fetal head and body adjust to maternal pelvis by changes of position.

b) Adjustments are known as cardinal movements, or mechanisms of labor.
  (1) Descent: Biparietal diameter of fetal head enters the pelvic inlet in occipitotransverse or oblique position.
  (2) Engagement: Biparietal diameter of fetal head (greatest transverse diameter) is at or passes the pelvic inlet.
  (3) Flexion: Neck bends so that chin touches sternum; suboccipitobregmatic diameter (smallest anteroposterior diameter) presents to pelvis.
  (4) Internal rotation: Head enters pelvis in occipitotransverse position, reaches pelvic floor, and rotates to occipitoanterior position.
  (5) Extension: Head lies beneath symphysis pubis; head extension follows, and face and chin are born.
  (6) External rotation: Head turns to the side (restitution); shoulders rotate to anteroposterior position in pelvis; shoulders and body are delivered (expulsion).

2. Fetal physiologic changes
  a) Fetal heart rate: Increased pressure on head frequently causes deceleration of heart rate during early part of contractions (see also section VI,A,2,d of this chapter for other fetal heart rate changes).
  b) Fetal movements
    (1) Breathing movements slow prior to onset of labor.
    (2) Gross body movements occur at 20–50 per hour.
    (3) Quiet and active sleep states occur.

V. Pain during labor and delivery

See text pages
_____

A. Mechanisms of pain: gate control theory
  1. Transmission of pain impulses is regulated by gating actions of central nervous system.
  2. Variations in pain perception are influenced by past experiences, distractions, thoughts, and feelings.
  3. Pain can be controlled by cutaneous stimulation and distraction and can be modified by activities controlled by the central nervous system.

B. Pain during stages of labor
  1. First stage: pain caused by dilatation of the cervix and uterine ischemia
    a) Discomfort is visceral.
    b) Pain is referred to lower abdominal wall and area over lower lumbar region and upper sacrum.

2. Second stage: pain caused by hypoxia of uterus, distention of vagina and perineum, pressure on adjacent structures
   a) Discomfort is somatic: Uterine contractions produce severe pain in lower back and suprapubic area.
   b) Discomfort may be local because of distention or laceration.
   c) Pain may also be referred to the back, flank, and thighs.
3. Third stage: pain caused by uterine contractions and cervical dilatation as placenta is expelled; discomfort similar to first stage

C. Factors affecting response to pain
   1. Knowledge and confidence gained through childbirth education
   2. Cultural influence on expression or repression of pain response (although stereotyping should be avoided)
   3. Maternal fatigue, sleep deprivation, and anxiety
   4. Personal significance and previous experience with pain
   5. Anticipation of pain
   6. Other sensations (stretching and pressure) misinterpreted as pain

D. General principles of pain management
   1. The goal of pain management is to produce maximal analgesia with minimal risk to client and fetus.
   2. The plan must take into consideration the effects of medication on the client, the contractions, and the fetus.
   3. Any disturbance of maternal homeostasis affects fetal environment.
   4. All systemic drugs cross placental barrier, and their actions depend on their rate of metabolism.
   5. The fetal blood-brain barrier is more permeable at birth.
   6. Effects on fetus are determined by maternal dosage, pharmacokinetics of drug, and route and timing of administration.
   7. Ideally, systemic medication is given to nullipara when cervix dilated 5–6 cm and to multipara when dilated 3–4 cm.
   8. Dosage is titrated until desired effect is achieved.

E. Methods of pain relief
   1. Nonpharmacologic pain relief
      a) Prepared childbirth methods (see Chapter 5, section VII,A)
         (1) Breathing techniques: specific breathing patterns that help the client maintain control during contractions and keep pressure of diaphragm off uterus
         (2) Relaxation exercises: progressive relaxation, touch relaxation, disassociation relaxation
         (3) Focusing attention on one object
         (4) Education regarding process of labor and delivery to decrease fear of unknown
      b) Effleurage: gentle, rhythmic stroking of abdomen during contractions
      c) Sensory stimulation: listening to music, applying heat and cold, smelling pleasant aromas, lower back massage or counter pressure during contractions

        d) Frequent position changes

        e) Transcutaneous electrical nerve stimulation (TENS): mild electrical current applied to lower back

    2. Systemic analgesics

        a) Use: during first stage of labor

        b) Administration: usually intravenous (IV) or intramuscular (IM)

        c) Advantages: have goal of providing maximum pain relief with minimal effects on fetus and uterus; decrease client's stress response

        d) Disadvantages: may cause depressive effects in client and fetus

        e) Types

            (1) Narcotic analgesics

                (a) Purpose: to inhibit transmission of pain impulses

                (b) Side effects: maternal mental clouding, respiratory depression, nausea, vomiting, orthostatic hypotension, urinary retention; fetal respiratory depression

                (c) Example: meperidine (Demerol)

            (2) Mixed narcotic agonist-antagonist compounds

                (a) Purpose: to inhibit transmission of pain impulses without causing respiratory depression

                (b) Side effect: will precipitate narcotic withdrawal in client who is narcotic addict

                (c) Examples: butorphanol tartrate (Stadol), nalbuphine (Nubain)

            (3) Analgesic potentiators (tranquilizers)

                (a) Purposes: to decrease anxiety and apprehension without prolonging labor, to potentiate narcotics, to prevent nausea and vomiting

                (b) Side effects: fetal hypotonia, lethargy, hypothermia; maternal respiratory depression when used with narcotics, hypotension

                (c) Examples: promethazine (Phenergan), hydroxyzine (Vistaril), diazepam (Valium)

            (4) Sedatives (barbiturates)

                (a) Purposes: to halt contractions of false labor or to allow client to rest and relax before onset of active labor

                (b) Side effects: maternal and fetal respiratory and vasomotor depression

                (c) Examples: secobarbital (Seconal), pentobarbital (Nembutal)

    3. Regional nerve blocks

        a) Use: during labor and vaginal delivery

        b) Administration: single injection or continuous infusion through catheter

c) Advantages: do not usually cause depressive effects in client; relief to blocked area is complete; client can be fully awake to push fetus down birth canal during labor

d) Disadvantages: may fail to take effect or may have incomplete effect; may have severe side effects such as respiratory or cardiac arrest and loss of consciousness; may cause toxic reaction; may cause nerve damage where catheter is placed

e) Types

   (1) Peridural block (lumbar epidural)

      (a) Purpose: to relieve pain during first and second stages of labor, during repair of episiotomy, and during cesarean section

      (b) Advantages: client fully awake; allows different blocking for each stage of labor; reflex urge to bear down is usually preserved

      (c) Disadvantages: breakthrough pain, sedation, pruritus, nausea, vomiting, hypotension, systemic toxic reaction

   (2) Spinal anesthesia (subarachnoid blockade)

      (a) Purpose: to relieve pain during cesarean section and during repair of episiotomy (not appropriate during labor because reflex urge to bear down is lost)

      (b) Advantages: fast-acting and easier to administer and uses smaller drug volume than peridural block

      (c) Disadvantages: high incidence of hypotension and greater potential for fetal hypoxia, drug reaction, total spinal anesthesia and paralysis of respiratory muscles, neurologic sequelae, spinal headache

   (3) Pudendal block

      (a) Purpose: to relieve pain during latter part of first stage of labor, second stage of labor, delivery, and episiotomy repair

      (b) Advantages: ease of administration, absence of maternal hypotension, preservation of reflex urge to bear down

      (c) Disadvantages: possible hematoma, perforation of rectum, trauma to sciatic nerve

   (4) Paracervical block

      (a) Purpose: to relieve pain of cervical dilatation during active phase of labor

      (b) Disadvantages: possibility of maternal systemic toxic reaction and hematoma; fetal bradycardia and decreased variability (therefore, not used often)

4. General anesthesia

   a) Use: for emergency cesarean section and surgical intervention due to obstetric complications

   b) Administration: IV, inhalation, or combination

   c) Advantages: total pain relief when immediate delivery or surgery is needed, such as for fetal distress or maternal hemorrhage

        d) Disadvantages: possibility of fetal respiratory depression, uterine relaxation, failed intubation, maternal vomiting and aspiration of vomitus

  F. Essential nursing care in pain management

    1. Nursing assessment: before administration of medicine

       a) History: Obtain information on allergies (especially anesthetic agents), smoking, neurologic and spinal disorders, presence of disease states, history of drug abuse, and usual methods of coping with pain.

       b) Interview: Determine the time and type of food last eaten; existing respiratory conditions; current drug use, including type, time of last use, and method of administration; unusual reactions to medication; maternal prenatal preparation and education; preferences for management of pain; time of onset of labor; status of membranes; complications of pregnancy; and problems since last seen by a physician.

       c) Fetal information: Determine gestational age, fetal response to labor, and results of fetal assessments (including fetal heart rate); palpate uterus to determine fetal size, position, and presentation.

       d) Maternal information: Ascertain character and status of labor, hydration status, and emotional reaction to the birthing process; perform vaginal examination; and have client empty bladder.

    2. Nursing assessment: after administration of medication

       a) Determine the level of pain relief and whether pain sensations return.

       b) Monitor for allergic or untoward reactions.

       c) Check blood pressure and fetal heart rate every 15 minutes after administration of regional anesthesia.

       d) Monitor contractions, cervical changes, and station of presenting part.

       e) Monitor fetal response, including changes in baseline, variability, accelerations, and possible decelerations.

       f) Monitor maternal emotional response.

    3. Nursing diagnoses

       a) Knowledge deficit related to expected sensation, client's role, options for pain management, and procedure for analgesia or anesthesia

       b) Situational low self-esteem related to negative perception of behavior

       c) Ineffective individual coping related to increased intensity and frequency of labor contractions

      d) High risk for altered fetal and maternal tissue perfusion related to effects of anesthesia or analgesia or maternal position

      e) High risk for maternal injury related to effects of anesthesia or analgesia on voluntary motor control or sensation

      f) Impaired urinary output related to effects of anesthesia

4. Nursing intervention

      a) Provide information about pain in the birthing process and methods to treat that pain.

      b) Explain procedures, such as administration of medication, positioning, and hydration; explain the importance of ongoing assessment (see Client Teaching Checklist, "Activities during Regional Anesthesia").

      c) Provide emotional support to client and support person; support decision about what type of analgesia to use.

      d) Administer medication (as ordered) to achieve maximum pain management with minimal risk to client and fetus.

      e) Monitor blood pressure and fetal heart rate; be alert for signs of maternal side effects and fetal distress.

✔ CLIENT TEACHING CHECKLIST ✔

Activities during Regional Anesthesia

Explanations to client:

✔ Blood pressure and pulse will be taken frequently during the administration; vital signs will be monitored every 15 minutes thereafter.

✔ You may feel a tingling or burning sensation as injection is given.

✔ Bladder will be assessed frequently, and you will be asked to void before anesthesia is administered.

✔ You will be intravenously hydrated prior to and throughout the anesthetic process.

✔ You will probably require intermittent catheterization after regional anesthesia has been administered.

✔ You may experience nausea, and an episode of vomiting may occur at any time during the infusion.

✔ You may feel sedated.

✔ The status of the fetus will be monitored continuously.

✔ You will be kept off your back to avoid decreased perfusion to both you and the fetus.

✔ Itching may develop during the infusion, and diphenhydramine may be given to minimize this side effect.

✔ Loss of sensation may decrease awareness of the urge to push; you will be assisted in coordinating pushing with contractions.

✔ Ambulation after delivery may be delayed until the anesthetic has worn off, perhaps taking several hours.

f) Hydrate adequately with IV fluids before, during, and after administration of regional anesthesia to minimize risk for hypotension.

g) Provide for safety needs of client with impaired mobility.

h) After regional anesthesia is administered, keep client off back to avoid vena caval compression.

i) Administer oxygen via face mask at 10–12 l/minute for fetal distress or maternal hypotension.

j) Collaborate with physician or nurse-anesthetist for medication orders to manage maternal hypotension and further pain.

k) Palpate client's bladder every 2 hours and encourage voiding. If regional anesthesia is being used, anticipate the need for catheterization.

5. Nursing evaluation

a) Nurse recognizes problems early and institutes corrective measures; client and fetus remain free of distress.

b) Client achieves adequate pain relief, is calmer, and feels more in control of birthing process.

c) Client understands the process of pain in labor and delivery, options for pain relief, and why it is necessary for the nurse to provide ongoing monitoring and evaluation.

d) Maternal and fetal vital signs stay within normal limits, normal labor continues, and no side effects are experienced.

See text pages

VI. Essential nursing care upon admission

A. Nursing assessment

1. Maternal assessment

a) History: Obtain name, age, attending physician, due date, available support system, previous illnesses, prenatal care record and problems, pregnancy data, prenatal education, results of special tests, blood type and Rh, list of medications and information on intrapartal risk factors, allergies, and food ingestion.

b) Physical examination: Assess general physical condition (including heart and lung sounds), vital signs, and blood pressure.

(1) Assess contractions (frequency, duration, intensity).

(2) Check amniotic fluid status: Nitrazine test determines the acidity or alkalinity of vaginal fluid (amniotic fluid pH 7–7.75).

(3) Check uterine activity using tocotransducer and/or palpation.

(4) Perform vaginal examination to determine:

(a) Degree of cervical dilatation: closed (0 cm) to completely dilated (10 cm).

      (b) Degree of effacement: 0% (thick) to 100% (thin).

      (c) Fetal position and station. (See Nurse Alert, "Vaginal Examination Warning.")

    (5) Ascertain need for pain medication; encourage use of nonpharmacologic methods first.

    (6) Check hydration status: skin turgor, mucous membranes, bladder distention, urine output.

  c) Lab work: Perform urinalysis (using dipstick to test for presence of protein in urine), hematocrit and hemoglobin, syphilis screening (VDRL), hepatitis (HBsAg) screening, and possible drug screening.

  d) Psychologic status: Observe emotions, support system (including marital status), verbal interaction, body language and posture, perceptual acuity, and energy level; note cultural background.

2. Fetal assessment

  a) Identify estimated date of delivery (EDD).

  b) Determine fundal height.

  c) Perform Leopold's maneuvers: 4 abdominal palpations that assess fetal position, lie, and presentation; done before initial vaginal examination.

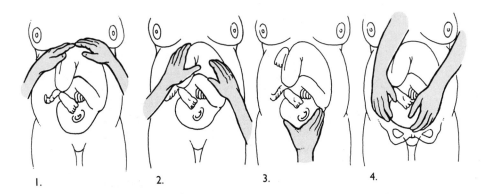

1.   2.   3.   4.

Figure 7-4
Leopold's Maneuvers

IV. Physiologic response to labor	V. Pain during labor and delivery	VI. Essential nursing care upon admission	VII. Essential nursing care: 1st stage of labor	VIII. Essential nursing care: 2nd stage of labor

       (1) Palpate upper abdomen with both hands: Head or buttocks should occupy fundus.

       (2) Palpate the sides of the abdomen with deep but gentle pressure: Determine location of fetal back and whether it is on right or left side.

       (3) Gently grasp the lower abdomen just above symphysis pubis: Determine what fetal part is lying above inlet.

       (4) Move fingers down sides of uterus toward pubis: Locate the cephalic prominence, or brow.

   d) Check fetal heart rate (FHR) through internal or external methods. (See Chapter 8, section III, for discussion of fetal distress.)

       (1) Baseline: normal 120–160 beats per minute (bpm), observed between contractions

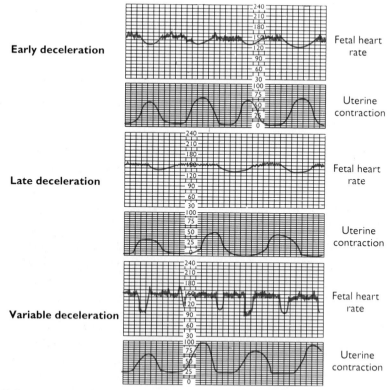

Figure 7-5
Fetal Heart Rate Patterns of Deceleration

(a) Bradycardia (<100 bpm or a drop of 20 bpm below baseline): can occur with progressive fetal acidosis, cord compression, placental separation

(b) Tachycardia (>160 bpm): can occur with breech presentation, maternal fever, fetal immaturity, fetal distress

(2) Variability: changes in FHR; described as minimal, moderate, marked

(a) Short-term: normal fluctuations in FHR between one heart beat and the next

(b) Long-term: normal fluctuations from baseline that occur in rhythmic cycles or waves; classified by number of beats per minute, from 0–>25

(c) Absence of variability: smooth (flat) baseline; sign of fetal distress, maternal drug use, or fetal sleep (can last up to 20 minutes)

(3) Periodic changes: transient accelerations or decelerations in fetal heart beat

(a) Accelerations: occur during fetal movement and contractions; classified as spontaneous, uniform, variable, rebound; usually considered a sign of fetal well-being

(b) Decelerations: described by their relation to onset and end of a contraction, their shape, and the severity of the drop (mild, moderate, severe)

  i) Early deceleration: normal response to head compression

  ii) Late deceleration: occurs after acme in response to uteroplacental insufficiency; ominous sign if uncorrectable

  iii) Variable deceleration: occurs at varying intervals in response to compression of umbilical cord (efforts should be made to eliminate the compression)

(4) Monitoring techniques

(a) Auscultation with fetoscope: to detect gross changes in fetal heart rate between, during, and after a contraction

(b) Electronic fetal monitoring (see Nurse Alert, "Indications for Electronic Fetal Heart Rate Monitoring")

  i) External (indirect) monitoring: ultrasound with transducer placed on woman's abdomen

  ii) Internal (direct) monitoring: electrode attached to fetal presenting part; may use fluid-filled intrauterine pressure catheter (IUPC) placed in uterine cavity to measure uterine activity and to correlate with FHR pattern; electrode and IUPC provide continuous data that are more accurate than data gathered through external monitoring

e) Perform fetal blood sampling, if needed: determines acid-base status of the fetus. Normal pH is ≥ 7.26.

B. Nursing diagnoses
   1. Anxiety related to hospital surroundings, labor and birth, possible loss of fetus
   2. Knowledge deficit related to expectations in labor, processes of labor, relaxation techniques, fetal monitoring procedures

C. Nursing intervention
   1. Provide reassurance to client as soon as she is admitted and throughout initial evaluation.
   2. Ask client to describe her expectations of the birthing process; provide information, as necessary, about labor, delivery, and relaxation techniques.
   3. Provide information about fetal monitoring: the equipment, when it is indicated, and what is involved in the monitoring procedures.
   4. Monitor fetal heart rate and identify patterns that require closer attention and treatment.
   5. Reassure client that her progress will be monitored closely and that nursing activities will focus on ensuring her and her fetus's well-being.

D. Nursing evaluation
   1. Client feels more comfortable and relaxed during the admission process.
   2. Client is knowledgeable about labor, delivery, and relaxation techniques.

! NURSE *ALERT* !

Indications for Electronic Fetal Heart Rate Monitoring

- Abnormal fetal heart rate on auscultation
- Passage of meconium or blood
- Decreased fetal movement
- Maternal fever, infection, disease
- Previous stillbirth
- Abnormal progression of labor
- Use of oxytocin, prostaglandin gel, regional anesthesia
- Prolonged or premature rupture of membranes
- Premature labor
- Prolapse of umbilical cord

NOTE: Electronic monitoring may be considered routine procedure by some physicians.

3. Client understands fetal monitoring equipment, when it is indicated, and what procedures may be involved.
4. Nurse closely monitors client and fetus and reports abnormalities promptly and accurately.
5. Client feels reassured that monitoring and nursing activities are effective in early identification and prevention of problems.
6. Client feels in control and has realistic expectations.

VII. Essential nursing care during the first stage of labor (see Chapter 8, section IV,A, for a discussion of induction when labor does not start spontaneously)

See text pages
_____

A. Nursing assessment
   1. General: Take blood pressure hourly and respiration rate, pulse, and temperature every 4 hours; clinical situations may dictate that vital signs be taken more frequently.
   2. Vaginal examination: Follow progress of labor; determine when to call certified nurse-midwife or physician; this examination is contraindicated if there is a history or signs of bleeding.
   3. Uterine contractions
      a) Monitor for frequency, duration, and intensity.
      b) Note changes in character as labor progresses: As client approaches transition, contractions get stronger, last about 60 seconds, and occur at 2- to 3-minute intervals, with uterus relaxing completely after each contraction.
      c) Determine level of pain and client's ability to use breathing and relaxation techniques effectively.
   4. Rupture of membranes: If membranes rupture, check fetal heart rate; then check fluid for color, odor, and amount.
   5. Fetal heart rate: Assess every 15 minutes during active phase of labor; assess before ambulation, enema administration, artificial rupture of membranes, and administration of analgesia or anesthesia.

B. Nursing diagnoses
   1. Fluid volume deficit related to decreased fluid intake
   2. Ineffective family coping related to client being in pain
   3. Alteration in comfort related to uterine contractions
   4. Self-care deficit related to immobility during labor
   5. Ineffective individual coping related to loss of control of bodily functions
   6. Altered placental tissue perfusion related to maternal position

C. Nursing intervention
   1. Provide ice chips or sips of clear fluids, as needed; maintain parenteral intake at 125 ml/hour.
   2. Encourage support person's participation; keep client and support person up to date on progress of labor.

3. In latent phase:
    a) Rub back and apply cool cloth to forehead.
    b) If client not on monitor, encourage ambulation and suggest frequent position changes; discourage supine position because uteroplacental perfusion is diminished.
    c) Encourage support person's involvement with breathing techniques during contractions.
    d) Provide information about discomfort:
        (1) It is intermittent and of limited duration.
        (2) Rest is necessary between contractions.
        (3) Distracting activities may prove helpful.
4. Change bed linens and gown; keep perineal area clean and dry.
5. Assist client and support person to focus on breathing and relaxation measures.
6. Support client's decision on pain medications.
7. Offer bedpan or help client to bathroom frequently.
8. Perform catheterization as needed for clients with regional anesthesia.
9. Check maternal vital signs regularly; attach fetal monitor or use fetoscope; check fetal heart rate for baseline, accelerations, variability, and decelerations.
10. Reposition client as needed to obtain optimal fetal heart rate pattern.
11. Review contraction and fetal heart rate patterns to determine need to reposition or need for further intervention.
12. Report presence of meconium-stained amniotic fluid to physician or nurse-midwife.

D. Nursing evaluation
    1. Client remains well-hydrated; fluid intake and output are within normal limits.
    2. Client has increased comfort through the use of self-comfort measures, administration of appropriate analgesia, and support from nurse and support person.
    3. Client and support person are reassured of the progress of labor.
    4. Fetus shows no signs of distress and has reassuring fetal heart rate measurements; maternal vital signs are within normal limits; labor progresses smoothly.
    5. Nurse recognizes problems early and institutes corrective measures; client and fetus remain free of distress.

VIII. Essential nursing care during the second stage of labor

See text pages
_____

A. Nursing assessment
 1. Be alert for signs that suggest onset of second stage of labor.
  a) Sudden appearance of sweat on upper lip
  b) Sudden increase in show, which is more blood-tinged
  c) Episode of vomiting
  d) Increase in apprehension or irritability
  e) Beginning of involuntary bearing-down efforts
  f) Rupture of membranes
  g) Change in pitch of voice (low, grunting sounds)
  h) Complaints of rectal and perineal pressure
 2. Perform vaginal examination to determine appropriateness of bearing down.
  a) Confirm complete dilatation of cervix (10 cm).
  b) Confirm descent of presenting part to introitus.
 3. Assess status of contractions (frequency, duration, intensity).
 4. Assess maternal physical status.
  a) Take pulse and blood pressure.
  b) Continue to monitor client's labor.
  c) Note presence of amnesia between contractions.
 5. Monitor fetal response and fetal heart rate: mild, brief bradycardias and early decelerations occur in 90% of women.
 6. Check amniotic fluid for meconium staining, odor, and amount.
 7. Assess client's and support person's coping status.

B. Nursing diagnoses
 1. Alteration in comfort: increased pain related to fetal position and contraction
 2. Ineffective individual coping related to physical exhaustion
 3. Anxiety related to unknown outcome of labor and possible loss of control
 4. Fatigue related to expenditure of energy during labor

C. Nursing intervention
 1. Continue to provide comfort measures of positioning, mouth care, clean and dry bedding, and a quiet environment.
 2. Position client for pushing; encourage complete rest between contractions.
 3. Instruct client on bearing-down positions and techniques (e.g., semi-Fowler, sitting, squatting, lateral). (See Client Teaching Checklist, "Methods for Bearing Down.")
 4. Continue to monitor contraction and fetal heart rate patterns to determine need for intervention.
 5. Continue providing psychosocial support in the form of reassurance and coaching; encourage support person to continue support.
 6. Give brief, explicit directions because client may fall asleep between contractions.

7. Prepare for delivery.
   a) Observe for perineal bulging and anal orifice dilatation.
   b) Transfer to delivery room with bed's side rails up or prepare delivery bed.
   c) Move client onto delivery bed between contractions.
   d) Position client for anesthesia and/or delivery.
   e) Explain all procedures and equipment to client and support person.
   f) Prep perineal area: clean the vulva and surrounding area.
8. Assist with delivery; support client during episiotomy.
   a) Crowning: widest part of fetal head distends the vulva just before birth; episiotomy usually done at this time to minimize soft tissue damage
   b) Ritgen maneuver: helps control delivery of head; forward pressure applied to fetal chin with one hand and downward pressure applied to occiput with other hand
   c) Bulb syringe: used to suction mouth and nose
   d) Delivery of body: anterior shoulder delivered, followed by posterior shoulder
9. Clamp the cord using 2 Kelly clamps; cut between the clamps before pulsations cease.
10. Facilitate family bonding.

D. Nursing evaluation
   1. Client maintains stable vital signs.
   2. Fetus maintains stable heart rate.
   3. Client pushes effectively and continues using breathing and relaxation techniques between contractions.
   4. Support person is actively involved and is able to provide reassurance and assistance during contractions.

✔ CLIENT TEACHING CHECKLIST ✔

Methods for Bearing Down

Explanations to client:

✔ Push only with the urge to push.
✔ Use abdominal muscles.
✔ Use short pushes of no longer than 6–7 seconds.
✔ Push approximately 3–5 times during each contraction.
✔ Push with an open glottis and slight exhale.

5. Client is safely transported to delivery room.
6. Client experiences a decrease in pain after anesthesia/analgesia is administered.
7. Client and support person understand delivery room procedures and equipment.
8. Client positions herself appropriately for birth and delivers a healthy infant.
9. Nurse recognizes problems early and institutes corrective measures; client and fetus remain free of distress.

IX. Essential nursing care during the third and fourth stages of labor (see Chapter 11 for additional information on postpartum nursing care)

See text pages
_____

A. Nursing assessment
   1. Monitor placental separation.
      a) Ascertain height and consistency of fundus immediately after delivery of infant.
      b) Observe for signs of separation.
         (1) Firm uterine contractions
         (2) Change in uterine shape from discoid to globular ovoid
         (3) Protrusion of umbilical cord from vagina (indicating placental descent)
         (4) Sudden gush of dark blood from vagina
   2. Determine need for oxytocics or prostaglandin to stimulate uterine contraction, promoting hemostasis.
   3. Monitor maternal physical status.
      a) Cardiac output should increase after delivery.
      b) Pulse should slow and blood pressure should return to prelabor levels.
      c) Bleeding should be minimal.
      d) Potential for rupture of preexisting cerebral aneurysm and pulmonary amniotic fluid emboli increases.
      e) Uterine fundus should contract to prevent hemorrhage.
   4. Assess level of pain resulting from episiotomy.
   5. Assess the newborn (see Chapter 9).

B. Nursing diagnoses
   1. Knowledge deficit related to procedure for delivery of placenta
   2. Fatigue related to energy expenditure during labor
   3. Alteration in comfort related to perineal lacerations
   4. Family coping: potential for growth related to changes in family structure
   5. Risk for altered uterine tissue perfusion related to uterine atony

C. Nursing intervention
   1. Describe the process involved in placental separation and expulsion.
   2. Instruct client to push when signs of separation have occurred.
   3. Administer oxytocic or prostaglandin if ordered and indicated.

4. Provide support and information to client regarding episiotomy repair and related pain relief and self-care measures.
5. To relieve pain of episiotomy, apply ice pack for 20–30 minutes after birth; remove for 30 minutes; reapply.
6. Clean and help client into comfortable position; assist with transfer to recovery area.
7. Encourage client to void.
8. Encourage bonding between parents and newborn; provide private environment for couple's first moments with infant; encourage breastfeeding if this is desired feeding method.
9. Monitor vital signs every 15 minutes for 1 hour, then every 30 minutes for next hour, then every hour for 2 hours.
10. Check perineal area daily to assess healing of episiotomy.
11. Monitor for return of sensation and ability to void if regional anesthesia was used.

D. Nursing evaluation
1. Client understands placental separation and her part in accomplishing it.
2. Client's placenta is delivered intact.
3. Client's uterus is firm; blood loss is less than 500 ml.
4. Client maintains stable vital signs.
5. Client is able to void.
6. Client is more comfortable and relaxed.
7. Couple have opportunity to bond with their new baby.
8. Breastfeeding is initiated if desired.

1. The fetal lie that allows the fetus to move through the birth canal most easily is:

   a. Transverse.
   b. Longitudinal.
   c. Perpendicular.
   d. Oblique.

2. Which of the following is a favorable vertex presentation?

   a. LOA
   b. RMA
   c. LSP
   d. RScA

3. The nurse is using Leopold's maneuvers to assess fetal position. The third Leopold's maneuver assesses the:

   a. Fetal part occupying the fundus.
   b. Fetal part lying above the pelvic inlet.
   c. Position of the fetal back.
   d. Location of cephalic prominence.

4. Sarah Anderson, nullipara, is admitted to the labor room with contractions every 3–5 minutes and lasting 45–60 seconds. She appears somewhat anxious and states that she is quite nauseated. Sarah is most likely in what phase of labor?

   a. Latent phase
   b. Active phase
   c. Transition phase
   d. Pushing phase

5. Sarah's membranes rupture spontaneously. The nurse's first action should be to:

   a. Assess fetal heart tones (FHT).
   b. Provide a clean gown and bed linen.
   c. Assess fetal station.
   d. Check color and amount of fluid.

6. When Sarah is dilated 5 cm, she asks for medication for pain. The nurse's best response is:

   a. "It's too early in your labor; medication will slow your labor."
   b. "Try to wait until you really need it."

   c. "I'll check your health care provider's medication order to see what I can give you."
   d. "Perhaps a change in position will make you more comfortable."

7. When Sarah is dilated 10 cm, she begins to push with each contraction. To help Sarah have effective pushing, the nurse should encourage her to:

   a. Push throughout the entire contraction.
   b. Chest-breathe with the contraction.
   c. Pant and blow during the contraction.
   d. Push for 6–7 seconds, 3–5 times during each contraction.

8. Sarah's diet order is sips of clear liquid and ice chips only. The primary reason for this is to:

   a. Prevent aspiration of stomach contents.
   b. Prevent fluid overload throughout labor.
   c. Accommodate the delayed gastric emptying associated with labor.
   d. Decrease urinary output and frequent urination.

9. Annette, multipara, is dilated 8 cm and is working hard to maintain control during her contractions. She reports that she feels light-headed and has a tingling sensation in her fingers. The nurse should:

   a. Change client's position.
   b. Assess fetal heart tones.
   c. Have client breathe into a paper bag.
   d. Administer oxygen.

10. Margaret, primigravida, is dilated 6 cm and is to receive a lumbar epidural anesthesia. A major advantage in using this method during labor is that it:

    a. Provides total pain relief at each stage.
    b. Prevents nausea and vomiting.
    c. Prevents maternal hypotension.
    d. Allows different pain blocking for each stage.

11. A client received an episiotomy during delivery. To facilitate the achievement of the goal "Client will state a decrease in episiotomy pain," the nurse should during the first half hour after birth:

   a. Offer warm blankets.
   b. Encourage client to void.
   c. Apply an ice pack to episiotomy.
   d. Offer a warm sitz bath.

12. Which of the following observations indicates that the placenta has separated?

   a. Cessation of all uterine contractions
   b. Change in uterine shape from discoid to globular
   c. A drop in maternal blood pressure
   d. Cessation of umbilical cord pulsations

ANSWERS

1. **Correct answer is b.** A longitudinal lie means that the long axis of the fetus is parallel to the woman's long axis. This facilitates passage through the birth canal.

   a. A transverse lie cannot be delivered vaginally.
   c. Perpendicular would be the same as transverse lie.
   d. An oblique lie means that the fetal long axis forms an acute angle in relation to maternal axis.

2. **Correct answer is a.** The left occipitoanterior (LOA) is a common and favorable vertex presentation.

   b. RMA is right mentoanterior, which is a face presentation.
   c. LSP is left sacroposterior, which is a breech presentation.
   d. RScA is right scapuloanterior, which is a shoulder presentation.

3. **Correct answer is b.** The third maneuver is done by gently grasping the lower abdomen just above the symphysis pubis. This is done to determine what fetal part is lying above the inlet.

   a. The first maneuver identifies the fetal part, head or buttocks, which should occupy the fundus.
   c. The second maneuver identifies the location of fetal back, whether it is on the right or left side.
   d. The fourth position identifies the location of a cephalic prominence, or brow.

4. **Correct answer is b.** The active phase of the first stage of labor is characterized by contractions every 3–5 minutes, lasting up to 60 seconds. Maternal response includes increasing anxiety, nausea, vomiting, and pain.

   a. During the latent phase of the first stage of labor, the uterine contractions are established and occur every 15–30 minutes, lasting 15–30 seconds. Women are usually able to cope with the discomfort.
   c. During the transition phase of the first stage of labor, contractions occur every 2–3 minutes and may last up to 90 seconds. Women become more internally directed, and anxiety increases. Pain is most acute.
   d. The pushing phase occurs during the second stage of labor. The woman has the urge to bear down. This stage begins when the cervix is completely dilated and ends with the birth of the baby.

5. **Correct answer is a.** After rupture of membranes, it is important to assess FHT. With the gush of water, there is a possibility of cord prolapse, resulting in a decrease in FHT and fetal distress.

   b. A clean gown and linens should be provided after monitoring fetal tones.
   c. Assessment of fetal station is not necessary as a result of rupture of membranes.
   d. Assessment of color and amount of fluid will help identify potential fetal distress (e.g., if the fluid is meconium-stained). However, FHT should be assessed first as it is a direct assessment of the fetus.

6. Correct answer is c. Physicians generally write medication orders to encompass parameters during the stages of labor.

a. Sarah's labor is well-established; medication would not slow labor at this point.
b. This is an inappropriate response because pain is whatever the client says it is.
d. Although it is true that position changes can enhance comfort, Sarah asked for pain medication.

7. Correct answer is d. To achieve effective pushing, the client should use abdominal muscles and push with the urge to push. She should not hold her breath for prolonged periods because this can diminish oxygen to the fetus. Pushing for 6–7 seconds, 3–5 times during a contraction, will be effective.

a. Pushing throughout an entire contraction requires the woman to hold her breath for a prolonged time; thus, fetal hypoxia could occur.
b. Slow chest breathing is effective during latent and active phases of the first stage of labor. However, it is not effective during the second stage.
c. Panting and blowing would be used if the client is trying to control the urge to push.

8. Correct answer is c. During labor, the gastrointestinal motility and absorption of food decrease. As a result, the woman in labor should have only ice chips or sips of clear liquids.

a. Aspiration is not normally a concern in labor. Should the client need a general anesthetic, it would be a significant issue.
b. Fluid overload is not a normal physiologic occurrence during labor.
d. A woman in labor needs to continue to have normal urinary output.

9. Correct answer is c. Annette is experiencing hyperventilation as she shows signs of respiratory alkalosis. This may be overcome by having client breathe into a paper bag. This enables her to rebreathe carbon dioxide.

a. A change in position would not help hyperventilation.
b. If the hyperventilation is not corrected, there may be a subsequent change in fetal heart tones.
d. Oxygen is not the required aspect. With hyperventilation, the client needs to rebreathe the carbon dioxide and replace the bicarbonate ion.

10. Correct answer is d. A lumbar epidural allows for incremental dosing to achieve a sensory block during the first and second stages of labor, during episiotomy repair, and during a cesarean section.

a. There is no guarantee that a lumbar epidural will provide total pain relief. In fact, one of its disadvantages is breakthrough pain.
b. Nausea and vomiting may be a side effect of using a lumbar epidural.
c. Maternal hypotension is one of the most frequent complications of a lumbar epidural.

11. Correct answer is c. Applying ice immediately will decrease pain and swelling at the episiotomy site.

a and **b.** Warm blankets and encouraging client to void may increase client comfort but do not affect episiotomy pain.
d. A sitz bath will be beneficial later. The first choice of treatment is an ice pack.

12. Correct answer is b. A change in the uterine shape from discoid to globular indicates that the placenta has separated.

a. Uterine contractions continue even after separation of placenta.
c. There should be no drop in maternal blood pressure as placental separation occurs.
d. Umbilical cord pulsations are stopped prior to placental separation with the clamping of the cord.

8

High-Risk Conditions and Complications during Labor and Delivery

NURSING HIGHLIGHTS

1. The 4 P's of labor (powers, passageway, psyche, passenger) work in complex harmony during childbirth; problems with any 1 or a combination of these labor essentials can cause dystocia.
2. Complicated labor causes enormous stress for the client and support person.
3. Nurse can help client and support person cope with stress by providing emotional and physical support.
4. Nurse should be supportive and reassuring but realistic throughout complicated labor and delivery.
5. Nurse must have thorough knowledge of normal childbirth process in order to detect abnormal variation.

6. Fetal or maternal distress requires rapid clinical assessment and prompt intervention to prevent serious sequelae or death.

7. Nursing care during obstetric interventions focuses on client education and the provision of emotional support.

GLOSSARY

amniotomy—artificial rupture of the amniotic membranes

breech presentation—fetal presentation in which buttocks and/or lower extremities enter the pelvis first

caput succedaneum—swelling of tissue on fetal head caused by pressure as it presents during labor

catecholamines—hormones produced in response to stress; in excessive amounts, have negative effect on labor

cephalopelvic disproportion—disproportion between size of pelvis and size of fetal head; causes dystocia

complete breech presentation—fetus presenting with legs folded on thighs and thighs flexed on abdomen

dystocia—painful, prolonged, or otherwise difficult birth because of mechanical or uterine factors

external version—turning fetus in uterus to change presenting part

frank breech presentation—fetal buttocks presenting with hips flexed and thighs against abdomen

incomplete breech presentation—1 or both fetal feet or knees presenting

ischial tuberosities—bony prominences on either side of maternal pelvic outlet

x-ray pelvimetry—measurement of pelvic dimensions using x-rays

ENHANCED OUTLINE

I. Dystocia

See text pages
_____

A. Maternal causes
   1. Powers
      a) Primary dysfunctional labor: abnormal uterine contractions that prevent normal progression of labor
         (1) Hypertonic labor patterns: painful, uncoordinated contractions; ineffective in causing dilatation and effacement
            (a) Occurrence: latent phase of labor, most often in nullipara and postterm pregnancies
            (b) Causes: stimulation of contractions from 2 or more pacemakers, disrupting fundal dominance of contractions; contributing factors of extreme anxiety, fear of unknown

    (c) Risks

        i) Maternal: extreme pain; discouragement and frustration

        ii) Fetal: fetal distress with excessive molding of head

    (d) Medical therapy: Arrest uterine activity and establish a more effective labor pattern with bed rest and sedation (oxytocin is contraindicated).

    (e) Nursing assessment

        i) Evaluate relationship between pain, intensity of contraction, and degree of dilatation and effacement.

        ii) Determine if anxiety is having harmful effect; check for changes in blood pressure, pulse, and level of consciousness.

    (f) Nursing diagnoses

        i) Anxiety related to slow progress of labor

        ii) High risk for ineffective individual coping related to ineffectiveness of relaxation techniques

        iii) Fatigue related to inability to relax

        iv) High risk for fetal distress related to decreased placental perfusion

    (g) Nursing intervention

        i) Provide comfort measures such as positioning, mouth care, and clean linens; encourage ambulation, if tolerated.

        ii) Reassure client and support person; provide environment for relaxation, and help them focus on breathing techniques.

        iii) Provide information on hypertonic labor pattern and fetal implications.

        iv) Provide sedation as ordered and indicated.

        v) Monitor fetus closely to detect possible distress.

    (h) Nursing evaluation

        i) Client experiences more effective labor pattern.

        ii) Client and support person understand hypertonic labor patterns.

        iii) Client has decreased anxiety and increased comfort.

        iv) Client gives birth to healthy infant.

  (2) Hypotonic labor patterns: contractions that decrease in frequency and intensity; slowing dialation and fetal descent

    (a) Occurrence: active phase of first stage of labor (after at least 4 cm of dilatation)

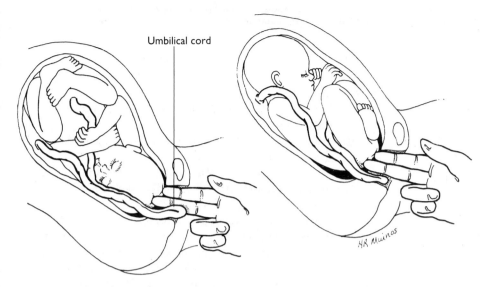

Figure 8-1
Removing Pressure from the Prolapsed Umbilical Cord

    (b) Causes: overstretching of uterine fibers, effects of
        sedation in early labor, possible cephalopelvic
        disproportion, fetal malposition
    (c) Risks
       i) Maternal: discouragement and anxiety, uterine
          infection because of prolonged labor, postpartal
          hemorrhage due to uterine atony
      ii) Fetal: tachycardia and sepsis
    (d) Medical therapy: Stimulate labor with oxytocin and
        amniotomy; perform cesarean section if labor does not
        resume.
    (e) Nursing assessment
       i) Check adequacy of pelvic measurements and
          gestational age.
      ii) Monitor for signs and symptoms of infection and
          dehydration (see Nurse Alert, "Signs of Infection").
      iii) Evaluate coping mechanisms of client and support
          person.
      iv) Encourage ambulation, if possible.
   (f) Nursing diagnoses
       i) High risk for fluid volume deficit related to
          prolonged labor and restricted fluid intake
      ii) High risk for infection related to prolonged rupture
          of membranes
      iii) Potential for maternal or fetal distress related to use
          of oxytocin
      iv) Potential for fetal distress related to amniotomy

 (g) Nursing intervention
   i) Monitor fluid intake and output and bladder distention.
   ii) Look for chills and changes in characteristics of amniotic fluid.
   iii) Monitor maternal vital signs, uterine contractions, and fetal heart rate (fetal scalp electrode may be necessary).
   iv) Provide information and support to client and support person.
   v) Provide comfort measures and promote relaxation.
   vi) Administer oxytocin according to protocol and monitor action of oxytocin (see Nurse Alert, "Maternal Danger Signs during Oxytocin Infusion").

 (h) Nursing evaluation
   i) Client has balanced fluid intake and output and does not show signs of infection.
   ii) Client and support person understand hypotonic labor pattern.
   iii) Maternal and fetal vital signs remain stable.
   iv) Deviations of client from normal labor pattern with oxytocin or amniotomy are noted, and appropriate interventions are made.
   v) Client gives birth to healthy infant.

 (3) Precipitous labor: extremely rapid labor (less than 3 hours)
  (a) Occurrence: onset of labor, often in multipara pregnancies

---

! NURSE *ALERT* !

Signs of Infection

- Fever
- Shaking chills
- Change in character of vaginal discharge
 —Odor
 —Color
 —Thickness

    (b) Causes: low resistance of maternal tissues, exceptionally strong contractions, oxytocin overdose, history of rapid labor, cocaine abuse, or small fetus in vertex position

    (c) Risks

        i) Maternal: perineal lacerations, uterine rupture, postpartal hemorrhage, amniotic fluid embolism

        ii) Fetal: cerebral trauma and hypoxia

    (d) Medical therapy

        i) Monitor client and fetus closely.

        ii) Possibly administer tocolytic agents such as magnesium sulfate ($MgSO_4$).

        iii) Prepare for emergency birth.

    (e) Nursing assessment

        i) Monitor contraction pattern and cervical changes.

        ii) Monitor fetal response to contractions.

        iii) Monitor maternal vital signs.

    (f) Nursing diagnoses

        i) Pain related to rapid labor

        ii) Ineffective individual coping related to contraction pattern and precipitous birth

        iii) Potential for fetal distress related to decreased placental perfusion

        iv) Potential for maternal injury related to rapid progression of labor

    (g) Nursing intervention

        i) Observe perineum at frequent intervals.

        ii) Provide comfort measures, encourage rest, and administer sedatives as ordered.

        iii) Assist client with appropriate breathing techniques (if birth is imminent, panting or blowing with each contraction).

        iv) Remain with client and provide reassurance.

        v) Provide hydration with IV line.

        vi) Prepare for emergency delivery.

         (h) Nursing evaluation

            i) Client is more comfortable and uses breathing measures to slow delivery.

            ii) Client and fetus remain in stable condition.

            iii) Deviations of client from normal labor pattern are noted, and appropriate interventions are made.

            iv) Client gives birth to healthy infant.

    (4) Prolonged labor: slow dilatation of cervix and lengthy labor (more than 24 hours)

         (a) Occurrence: first stage of labor

         (b) Causes: cephalopelvic disproportion (CPD), malposition, dysfunctional labor patterns, cervical dystocia

         (c) Risks

            i) Maternal: unproductive pain, exhaustion, infection, hemorrhage

            ii) Fetal: asphyxia, infection, cord prolapse, head bruising or trauma

         (d) Medical therapy: Administer prostaglandin gel to soften and efface cervix, then oxytocin if indicated; perform an amniotomy.

         (e) Nursing assessment

            i) Monitor contraction patterns closely.

            ii) Monitor fetal response to contractions: Check fetal heart rate, and check amniotic fluid for presence of meconium.

            iii) Calculate fluid intake and output; check urine for presence of ketones.

         (f) Nursing diagnoses

            i) High risk for infection related to increased need for invasive assessments

            ii) High risk for ineffective individual coping related to prolonged labor

            iii) Potential for maternal or fetal distress related to effects of prostaglandin gel and oxytocin

            iv) High risk for fluid volume deficit related to length of labor and restricted fluid intake

         (g) Nursing intervention

            i) Monitor for signs of infection.

            ii) Provide comfort measures such as sponge baths, position changes, and back rubs.

            iii) Help client focus on breathing and relaxation techniques.

            iv) Maintain fluid balance.

    v) Administer prostaglandin gel and oxytocin according to protocol.
    vi) Monitor contractions and fetal heart rate pattern.
    vii) Perform vaginal exams as needed to monitor cervical and fetal changes.
  (h) Nursing evaluation
    i) Client remains free of infection.
    ii) Client avoids exhaustion, panic, and discouragement; client copes with prolonged labor.
    iii) Client maintains healthy fluid balance.
    iv) Deviations of client from normal labor pattern are noted, and appropriate interventions are made.
    v) Client gives birth to healthy infant.
b) Secondary dysfunctional labor: impaired bearing-down efforts that prevent normal progression of labor
  (1) Occurrence: second stage of labor (after cervix has reached 10 cm dilatation)
  (2) Causes: anesthesia, heavy analgesia, fatigue, pain, physical injury, position
  (3) Risks
    (a) Maternal: discouragement, frustration, exhaustion
    (b) Fetal: asphyxia
  (4) Medical therapy
    (a) Allow effects of analgesia/anesthesia to wear off.
    (b) Administer analgesia for pain.
    (c) Perform assisted vaginal or cesarean delivery.
  (5) Nursing assessment
    (a) Observe effectiveness of pushing technique.
    (b) Monitor emotional status of client.
    (c) Monitor fetal heart rate pattern.
  (6) Nursing diagnoses
    (a) Potential for ineffective individual coping related to ineffectiveness of pushing effort and exhaustion
    (b) Potential for fetal distress related to prolonged labor
    (c) High risk for uterine atony related to prolonged labor
  (7) Nursing intervention
    (a) Provide comfort measures.
    (b) Reassure client and support person.
    (c) Assist client in finding more effective pushing technique and position (e.g., semi-Fowler, sitting, squatting, lateral).
    (d) Encourage complete rest between contractions.
    (e) Continue to monitor contraction and fetal heart rate pattern.
  (8) Nursing evaluation
    (a) Client experiences increased comfort.
    (b) Client avoids exhaustion, discouragement, and frustration.

          (c) Client pushes effectively.

          (d) Client maintains healthy fluid balance.

          (e) Client gives birth to healthy infant.

2. Passageway

  a) Pelvic dystocia: pelvic abnormality that results in cephalopelvic disproportion (CPD) and which prevents normal progression of labor

    (1) Types of abnormalities of bony pelvis

      (a) Contracted pelvis: inadequate major diameters; categorized by location

        i) Pelvic inlet: anteroposterior diameter <10 cm

        ii) Midpelvis: distance between ischial spines <9 cm

        iii) Pelvic outlet: distance between ischial tuberosities <8 cm

      (b) Unfavorable pelvic shapes: Android and platypelloid types predispose to CPD, as do some combinations of types.

    (2) Risks

      (a) Maternal: prolonged labor, premature rupture of membranes, uterine rupture

      (b) Fetal: cord prolapse, skull fracture, intracranial hemorrhage

    (3) Medical therapy

      (a) Evaluate pelvic diameters (x-ray pelvimetry, manual examination, magnetic resonance imaging).

      (b) Continue labor with careful monitoring (trial labor).

      (c) Perform assisted vaginal or cesarean delivery.

    (4) Nursing assessment

      (a) Determine adequacy of pelvis antepartally and intrapartally; report findings to physician.

      (b) Maintain high index of suspicion if labor is prolonged, dilatation and effacement are slow, and engagement of presenting part is delayed.

    (5) Nursing diagnoses

      (a) Knowledge deficit related to cephalopelvic disproportion

      (b) Fear related to unknown outcome of labor

    (6) Nursing intervention

      (a) Continue to monitor maternal and fetal well-being.

      (b) Chart progress of labor.

      (c) Change maternal position to increase pelvic diameters (sitting, squatting, or switching to other side).

        (d) Provide emotional support and reassurance.

        (e) Provide frequent reports on the progress of labor.

        (f) Provide information on cephalopelvic disproportion.

     (7) Nursing evaluation

        (a) Client understands cephalopelvic disproportion and possible alternative treatment plans.

        (b) Client verbalizes relief from fear and anxiety.

        (c) Client gives birth to healthy infant.

  b) Soft tissue dystocia: obstruction of fetal passage by anatomic abnormality other than bony pelvis

     (1) Causes: placenta previa, tumor, cervical edema, pathologic retraction ring (Bandl's ring)

     (2) Medical therapy (same as section I,A,2,a,3 of this chapter)

     (3) Essential nursing care (same as sections I,A,2,a,4–7 of this chapter)

3. Psyche

  a) Influences duration and character of labor

     (1) Fear, anxiety, and tension increase stress and cause release of catecholamines that can decrease uterine contractility.

     (2) Stress interferes with client's ability to work with her contractions.

     (3) Stress increases fatigue.

  b) Causes: pain, absence of support person, fear of unknown

  c) Nursing assessment

     (1) Monitor client's psychologic response to labor.

     (2) Determine client's level of stress.

     (3) Determine support person's level of anxiety.

     (4) Provide support.

     (5) Encourage relaxation.

  d) Nursing diagnoses

     (1) Ineffective individual coping related to anxiety and fear of the unknown

     (2) Ineffective family coping related to anxiety

  e) Nursing intervention

     (1) Reassure client and support person.

     (2) Create relaxed and private environment.

     (3) Encourage upright position (reduces the release of stress-related hormones).

     (4) Provide information on childbirth process.

     (5) Provide support person if needed.

  f) Nursing evaluation

     (1) Client and support person have reduced stress and are able to work together in promoting relaxation.

     (2) Client feels more in control of the childbirth process.

     (3) Client gives birth to healthy infant.

B. Fetal (passenger) causes
1. Fetal malposition
a) Persistent occipitoposterior: Fetal head enters pelvis with occiput directed diagonally posterior; fetal head must turn 135° in the process of internal rotation.
(1) Maternal risks: perineal laceration or extension of midline episiotomy
(2) Medical therapy
(a) Monitor progress of labor closely.
(b) Use forceps or manual rotation.
(c) Perform vaginal or cesarean delivery.
(3) Nursing assessment
(a) Assess client for intense back pain during first stage of labor.
(b) Monitor labor progress and cervical changes.
(4) Nursing diagnoses
(a) Pain related to occiput pressing on sacrum
(b) High risk for ineffective individual coping related to unanticipated outcome and slow progress in labor
(5) Nursing intervention
(a) Assist client to change positions frequently.
(b) Apply sacral pressure and perform back rubs.
(c) Provide support and reassurance to client and support person.
(d) Provide information on progress of labor.
(e) Encourage and instruct support person in providing comfort measures such as sponge bath, back rubs, and gentle distraction.
(6) Nursing evaluation
(a) Client experiences increased comfort.
(b) Client's coping abilities are strengthened; she and support person feel supported and reassured.
(c) Client gives birth to healthy infant.
b) Transverse arrest: Fetal head rotates incompletely; head arrests in transverse position.
(1) Risks
(a) Maternal: soft tissue damage
(b) Fetal: cerebral damage if condition is undetected
(2) Medical therapy
(a) Administer oxytocin.
(b) Use forceps or perform manual rotation (many spontaneously rotate).
(c) Perform vaginal or cesarean delivery.
(3) Essential nursing care (same as sections I,B,1,a,3–6)

2. Fetal malpresentation
  a) Breech presentations
    (1) Types: frank, complete, or incomplete (footling)
    (2) Risks
      (a) Maternal: perineal lacerations and postpartum infections
      (b) Fetal: increased mortality and morbidity related to congenital malformations and prematurity, cord prolapse, cerebral trauma
    (3) Medical therapy
      (a) Perform external version to convert breech to cephalic presentation if presenting part is not engaged.
      (b) Assess factors related to delivery methods (scoring systems developed to determine route of delivery).
      (c) Perform vaginal or cesarean delivery.
    (4) Nursing assessment
      (a) Determine breech presentation by palpation, ballottement, or auscultation for fetal heart rate.
      (b) Note passage of meconium after rupture of membranes.
      (c) Be alert for signs of prolapsed cord.
    (5) Nursing diagnoses
      (a) High risk for impaired fetal gas exchange related to compressed umbilical cord
      (b) Knowledge deficit related to breech presentation and associated complications
      (c) Fear related to unknown outcome
    (6) Nursing intervention
      (a) Closely monitor maternal and fetal well-being and be alert for signs of distress.
      (b) Educate client and support person on breech presentations, implications for delivery, and associated complications.
      (c) Provide reassurance.
      (d) Prepare client for delivery (either cesarean or vaginal).
    (7) Nursing evaluation
      (a) Nurse recognizes problems early and institutes corrective measures; client and fetus remain free of distress.
      (b) Client and support person verbalize understanding of the situation and are less fearful and anxious.
      (c) Client gives birth to healthy infant.
  b) Face and brow presentations
    (1) Risks
      (a) Maternal: vaginal lacerations and infection from prolonged labor
      (b) Fetal: facial ecchymosis and edema and caput succedaneum (face presentation)

  (2) Medical therapy
   (a) Deliver vaginally if labor is effective and pelvis is adequate.
   (b) Perform cesarean delivery if there is contracted pelvis or fetal distress.
  (3) Nursing assessment
   (a) Determine fetal position using Leopold's maneuvers.
   (b) During vaginal exam, attempt to palpate fontanels and nose.
   (c) Monitor fetal heart rate pattern.
  (4) Nursing diagnoses
   (a) Anxiety related to unknown outcome
   (b) Knowledge deficit related to face or brow presentation
   (c) High risk for injury to fetus related to pressure on fetal structures during birth process
   (d) High risk for fetal distress related to prolonged labor
  (5) Nursing intervention
   (a) Monitor progress of labor: contractions, changes in cervical dilatation and effacement, and fetal position.
   (b) Monitor fetal well-being; observe closely for signs of fetal distress, especially hypoxia. (Do not attach internal fetal electrode, as it may cause facial trauma.)
   (c) Prepare client and support person for possible fetal facial appearance; provide reassurance that swelling and bruising will resolve.
   (d) Provide information on face or brow presentation.
   (e) Prepare client for vaginal or cesarean delivery.
   (f) Provide reassurance to client and support person.
  (6) Nursing evaluation
   (a) Client and support person understand the implications and complications of face or brow presentation and are prepared for possible fetal facial abnormalities.
   (b) Client and fetus remain free of distress.
   (c) Client gives birth to healthy infant.
 c) Shoulder presentation (transverse lie)
  (1) Risks
   (a) Maternal: dysfunctional labor and uterine rupture
   (b) Fetal: prolapsed cord
  (2) Medical therapy
   (a) Perform external version for vaginal delivery if fetus is movable and client is not in active labor.
   (b) Perform cesarean birth if external version is not successful or indicated.

(3) Essential nursing care: Palpate to determine fetal position and presenting part; assess maternal and fetal vital signs; provide education and support to client and support person; prepare client for vaginal or cesarean birth.

3. Hydrocephalus: excessive accumulation of cerebrospinal fluid in fetal brain, causing cranial enlargement
    a) Risks
        (1) Maternal: breech presentations, obstructed labor, uterine rupture
        (2) Fetal: poor prognosis because of other congenital malformations, brain damage, infection
    b) Medical therapy: Select least traumatic birth route.
    c) Nursing assessment
        (1) Identify informational needs and emotional state of client and support person.
        (2) Provide support and reassurance.
    d) Nursing diagnoses
        (1) Knowledge deficit related to hydrocephalus
        (2) Anxiety related to unknown outcome
        (3) Anticipatory grieving related to knowledge of hydrocephalus
    e) Nursing intervention
        (1) Provide information on hydrocephalus, implications for delivery, and associated complications.
        (2) Assist during diagnostic procedures and explain or interpret results for client and support person.
        (3) Provide emotional support; encourage expressions of anxiety and grief due to newborn's congenital anomalies.
    f) Nursing evaluation
        (1) Client and support person receive adequate information and have their questions answered.
        (2) Client and support person feel supported in their anxiety and grief.

4. Prolapsed umbilical cord
    a) Types
        (1) Umbilical cord falls or is washed down through cervix into vagina.
        (2) Umbilical cord lies beside or just ahead of fetal presenting part (occult cord prolapse).
    b) Causes: breech presentation, transverse lie, unengaged presenting part, twin gestation, small fetal size, premature rupture of membranes
    c) Fetal risks: reduced circulation, fetal distress as cord is pressed between maternal pelvis and presenting part
    d) Medical therapy
        (1) Reduce compression: reposition client and lift fetal presenting part off cord.
        (2) Perform vaginal or cesarean delivery as soon as possible.

e) Nursing assessment
    (1) Identify client at risk for prolapsed cord.
    (2) Observe perineum and evaluate fetal heart rate pattern when presenting part not engaged and membranes rupture.
f) Nursing diagnoses
    (1) High risk for impaired gas exchange in fetus related to decreased blood flow
    (2) Fear related to unknown outcome
g) Nursing intervention
    (1) Closely monitor maternal and fetal status.
    (2) Prepare to institute emergency measures (see Nurse Alert, "Emergency Measures for Prolapsed Umbilical Cord").
    (3) Provide emotional support.
h) Nursing evaluation
    (1) Nurse recognizes problems early and institutes corrective measures; client and fetus remain free of distress.
    (2) Fetal heart rate pattern remains in normal range.
    (3) Client and support person feel supported.
    (4) Client gives birth to healthy infant.

II. Gestational problems

See text pages
_____

A. Premature rupture of membranes (PROM) (same as section II,E of Chapter 6)

B. Pregnancy-induced hypertension (PIH) (same as section II,A of Chapter 6)

C. Bleeding (hemorrhagic) problems
  1. Placenta previa (same as section II,D,1 of Chapter 6)
  2. Abruptio placentae (same as section II,D,2 of Chapter 6)
  3. Abdominal trauma
    a) Causes: automobile accidents (including decelerating injuries), falls, assault with penetrating injuries (gunshot or stab wounds)
    b) Risks
      (1) Maternal: uterine rupture, abruptio placentae, premature labor
      (2) Fetal: prematurity, hypoxia, mortality
    c) Medical therapy
      (1) Stabilize the injury and promote maternal and fetal well-being: ABCs (adequacy of *a*irway, presence of *b*reathing, *c*ardiovascular status).
      (2) Avoid supine hypotensive syndrome.
      (3) Treat maternal hypoxia and hypovolemia promptly.
      (4) Have cross-matched blood available.

    d) Nursing assessment
        (1) Determine maternal status (ABCs) and extent of injury.
        (2) Determine fetal status (fetal heart rate pattern and fetal movement).
        (3) Assess uterus for tenderness, tone, and contractions.
        (4) Check for vaginal bleeding or fluid leakage.
    e) Nursing diagnoses
        (1) High risk for injury related to maternal hypoxia, hemorrhage, cardiovascular collapse, brain or tissue damage
        (2) Pain related to effects of trauma
        (3) Fear related to danger to self and fetus
        (4) Knowledge deficit related to injuries and treatment
    f) Nursing intervention
        (1) Assist with emergency life-support measures.
        (2) Monitor maternal vital signs every 5–10 minutes.
        (3) Promote fetal well-being by having client lie on left side (reducing vena cava compression).
        (4) Monitor fetal heart rate pattern.
        (5) Observe for signs of preterm labor and abruptio placentae.
        (6) Provide information, support, and reassurance to client and family.
    g) Nursing evaluation
        (1) Patent airway is maintained; maternal vital signs and condition remain stable.
        (2) Fetal condition remains stable with normal heart rate and pattern.
        (3) Maternal trauma is treated.
        (4) Pain is adequately relieved.
        (5) Complications are detected and treated early.
        (6) Client and family understand consequences of injury and are able to express their feelings and concern, including grief if fetal death results.
        (7) Pregnancy continues, client recovers, and healthy term infant is delivered.

D. Preterm labor (see also Chapter 6, section II,F): labor initiated between 20 and 37 weeks
   1. Medical therapy when preterm labor cannot be suppressed
      a) Prepare for delivery or transport client to a tertiary care center.
      b) Avoid giving analgesics/anesthetics to prevent fetal respiratory depression at birth.
      c) Perform episiotomy, deliver head between contractions, and use forceps to protect head during vaginal birth.
      d) Perform cesarean delivery if fetus is in breech position.
   2. Nursing assessment
      a) Monitor fetal heart rate continuously.
      b) Chart fluid intake and output.
      c) Assess informational needs of client and support person.
      d) Assess labor progress.
   3. Nursing diagnoses
      a) Anxiety and fear related to unknown outcome
      b) Anticipatory grieving related to potential complications in premature newborn
      c) Knowledge deficit related to unexpected early labor
      d) Alteration in comfort related to uterine contractions
   4. Nursing intervention
      a) Provide information and answer questions.
      b) Maintain hydration with large-bore IV line.
      c) Provide supportive care.
      d) Provide comfort measures as in normal birth process (see Chapter 7, section V).
      e) Alert nursing personnel regarding anticipated delivery of high-risk infant.
   5. Nursing evaluation
      a) Client and support person verbalize an understanding of preterm labor.
      b) Client is able to cope with anxiety and fear.
      c) Client experiences increased comfort.
      d) Client and support person feel supported.
      e) Client gives birth to healthy infant.

E. Postdate pregnancy: pregnancy that extends past 42 weeks of gestation (or exceeds 294 days after first day of last menstrual period)
   1. Risks
      a) Maternal: prolonged labor process and increased incidence of operative (forceps delivery, episiotomy) and cesarean deliveries
      b) Fetal: hypoxia (placental circulation insufficiency), oligohydramnios (amniotic fluid deficiency), umbilical cord compression, macrosomia (>4000 g), asphyxia, meconium aspiration, mortality

2. Medical therapy
    a) Perform biophysical profile (BPP) and nonstress test weekly to determine fetal status (see Chapter 6, section IV,B, for description of biophysical tests).
    b) Possibly perform contraction stress test weekly to determine fetal status.
    c) Induce labor by 42 weeks or earlier according to results of BPP (a BPP of ≥8 is reassuring).
3. Nursing assessment
    a) Establish estimated date of delivery.
    b) Continuously monitor fetal heart rate pattern with electronic monitors.
    c) Check amniotic fluid for presence of meconium.
    d) Assess progress of labor and labor pattern.
4. Nursing diagnoses
    a) Knowledge deficit related to postdate pregnancy
    b) Fear related to unknown outcome
    c) High risk for fetal distress related to decreased placental perfusion
5. Nursing intervention
    a) Provide information and answer questions regarding postdate labor and its implications.
    b) Provide support to client and support person.
    c) Prepare for possible resuscitation of asphyxiated infant.
    d) Monitor closely to detect early onset of fetal distress.
6. Nursing evaluation
    a) Nurse recognizes problems early and institutes corrective measures; client and fetus remain free of distress.
    b) Client understands postdate labor and its implications.
    c) Client and support person feel supported.
    d) Client gives birth to healthy infant.

F. Multiple gestation
    1. Risks
        a) Maternal: uterine dysfunction due to overstretching, fetal malpresentation, preterm labor, abruptio placentae, hydramnios, pregnancy-induced hypertension
        b) Fetal: congenital anomalies, twin-to-twin transfusion syndrome (1 twin overperfused and the other underperfused), prematurity
    2. Medical therapy
        a) Monitor fetal and maternal status closely.
        b) Ready client for possible anesthesia; cross-matched blood should be available.
        c) Determine method of delivery.
        d) Delay use of oxytocin until first twin is delivered.
        e) Examine placentas after birth.
    3. Nursing assessment
        a) Monitor fetal heart rate patterns and uterine activity continuously.
        b) Determine family's level of preparation.

4. Nursing diagnoses
   a) Fear and ineffective individual coping related to uncertain labor and delivery
   b) Knowledge deficit related to implications and problems associated with multiple gestation
   c) High risk for impaired gas exchange related to decreased oxygenation secondary to cord compression or twin-to-twin transfusion
5. Nursing intervention
   a) Provide hydration with large-bore IV.
   b) Provide information about labor process and possible problems associated with multiple gestation.
   c) Prepare to receive 2 infants.
   d) Prepare to resuscitate 2 infants.
   e) Alert nursing personnel for arrival of twins.
   f) Provide support to client and support person and refer to community agencies, if necessary.
6. Nursing evaluation
   a) Nurse recognizes problems early and institutes corrective measures; client and fetuses remain free of distress.
   b) Client is knowledgeable about problems associated with multiple gestation and is able to cope with labor.
   c) Client gives birth to healthy infants.

See text pages

III. Fetal distress: fetal difficulty caused by insufficient oxygen supply

A. Causes
   1. Cord compression
   2. Uteroplacental insufficiency associated with placental abnormalities
   3. Preexisting maternal or fetal disease
   4. Uterine hyperstimulation from labor induction with prostaglandin gel or oxytocin

B. Signs (see Nurse Alert, "Signs of Fetal Distress")

C. Risks
   1. Maternal: increased psychologic stress, uterine rupture from uterine hyperstimulation
   2. Fetal: developmental delays (resulting from hypoxia), cerebral palsy, mortality

D. Medical therapy
   1. Change maternal position.
   2. Order oxygen by mask at 10–12 l/minute.

3. Institute electronic fetal monitoring.
4. Discontinue oxytocin if in use.
5. Provide tocolytic intervention with IV terbutaline for uterine hyperstimulation.
6. Expedite vaginal or cesarean delivery if labor does not progress and fetal distress continues.

E. Essential nursing care
 1. Nursing assessment
    a) Review prenatal history to anticipate possibility of fetal distress.
    b) Observe amniotic fluid for meconium (in vertex presentation).
    c) Be alert to changes in fetal heart rate pattern and fetal scalp pH and to reports by client of greatly increased or decreased fetal activity.
    d) Observe contraction pattern for hypertonic contractions.
 2. Nursing diagnoses
    a) Decreased cardiac output in fetus related to decreased uteroplacental perfusion
    b) Fear related to knowledge of fetal distress
 3. Nursing intervention
    a) Assist client to change position to relieve pressure on vena cava, including lowering head of bed (see Nurse Alert, "Emergency Measures for Prolapsed Umbilical Cord").
    b) Administer oxygen and increase fluid infusion rate.
    c) Discontinue oxytocin.
    d) Notify physician.
    e) Follow protocol for placing internal fetal monitor, if possible.
    f) Inform client of fetal status, explain treatment plan, and provide emotional support.
    g) Observe and record the signs of fetal distress.
    h) Prepare client for possible emergency vaginal or cesarean delivery.

4. Nursing evaluation
    a) Fetal distress is identified quickly and corrected.
    b) Client and support person feel supported and able to cope with situation.
    c) Fetal heart rate pattern returns to normal range.
    d) Client gives birth to healthy infant.

IV. Obstetric interventions

See text pages
_____

A. Induction of labor
    1. Definition: artificial initiation of uterine contractions before their spontaneous onset
        a) Indicated: preexisting maternal disease, pregnancy-induced hypertension, premature rupture of membranes, postdate pregnancy, fetal demise
        b) Elective: risk of precipitous delivery
    2. Prerequisite labor readiness factors
        a) Fetal maturity: assessed by ultrasound, fetal lung maturity tests, amniotic fluid studies
        b) Cervical status
            (1) Scoring system is used for predicting inducibility.
            (2) System evaluates dilatation, effacement, consistency, and fetal position and station.
            (3) Cervical status is most important criterion for successful induction.
    3. Medical therapy
        a) Determine any contraindications to induction.
        b) Apply prostaglandin gel to cervix.
        c) Perform amniotomy.
        d) Administer oxytocin by secondary line.
    4. Nursing assessment
        a) Assess maternal and fetal status.
        b) Perform vaginal examination to assess cervical status.
        c) Prior to each advancement of oxytocin infusion rate, check maternal blood pressure and pulse, fetal heart rate and reactivity, and status of contractions.
    5. Nursing diagnoses
        a) Knowledge deficit related to induction procedure
        b) Altered placental tissue perfusion related to potential for hypertonic contraction
        c) Pain related to uterine contractions

6. Nursing intervention
   a) Apply fetal and maternal electronic monitor.
   b) Explain to client the technique, rationale, and reactions to expect.
   c) Position client on her side; avoid supine position.
   d) Monitor maternal pulse and fetal heart rate every 15–20 minutes.
   e) Administer oxytocin according to protocol; be alert to danger signs (see Nurse Alert, "Maternal Danger Signs during Oxytocin Infusion").
   f) Provide comfort measures.
7. Nursing evaluation
   a) Nurse recognizes problems early and institutes corrective measures; client and fetus remain free of distress.
   b) Maternal and fetal vital signs stay within normal limits.
   c) Client and support person understand induction.
   d) Client establishes appropriate contraction pattern; fetal reactivity is within normal limits.
   e) Client gives birth to healthy infant.

B. Deliveries
   1. Cesarean delivery
      a) Definition: birth of infant through abdominal and uterine incision (usually low-segment)
      b) Indications: dystocia, placenta previa, prolapsed cord, previous cesarean (after considering vaginal birth after cesarean [VBAC]), breech and other malpresentations, fetal distress, herpes simplex virus type II
      c) Nursing assessment: preoperative
         (1) Obtain nursing history; perform physical examination and laboratory tests.
         (2) Evaluate client's readiness and understanding of procedure.
      d) Nursing diagnoses: preoperative
         (1) Knowledge deficit related to cesarean birth
         (2) Impaired gas exchange related to shallow breathing
         (3) Anxiety related to cesarean birth
         (4) Self-esteem disturbance related to inability to complete vaginal birth
      e) Nursing intervention: preoperative
         (1) Provide information on cesarean birth and describe preoperative procedure.
         (2) Encourage expression of feelings and provide support.
         (3) Establish large-bore IV line.
         (4) Insert Foley catheter.
         (5) Complete skin preparation.
         (6) See that consent forms have been signed.
      f) Nursing assessment: postoperative
         (1) Determine blood loss; normal upper limit is 1000 ml.
         (2) Monitor vital signs, including lochia and fundal checks.

        (3) Monitor fluid intake and output.

        (4) Determine degree of pain.

        (5) Observe bonding.

    g) Nursing diagnoses: postoperative

        (1) Pain related to incision and uterine involution

        (2) Altered tissue perfusion related to blood loss

        (3) Altered fluid and electrolyte balance related to fluid loss

        (4) Grieving related to inability to experience vaginal birth

        (5) High risk for altered parenting related to lack of early contact

    h) Nursing intervention: postoperative

        (1) Provide appropriate analgesia.

        (2) Assist in side-to-side turning, coughing, and deep breathing.

        (3) Assist with early ambulation, if indicated.

        (4) Monitor blood loss on surgical dressing and serial hemoglobin/hematocrit determinations.

        (5) Maintain balance of fluid and electrolytes with parenteral and oral replacement.

        (6) Provide routine postoperative and postpartum care (see Chapter 11 for postpartum care).

        (7) Encourage bonding.

    i) Nursing evaluation

        (1) Client and support person understand cesarean delivery procedure and why it is indicated.

        (2) Client and support person are able to express their feelings, especially of failure that vaginal birth is not possible.

        (3) Client understands postoperative and postpartum care; anxiety is lessened as she sees how she can participate.

        (4) Client feels comfortable postoperatively and has no complications.

        (5) Client and support person are able to interact with infant.

2. Forceps delivery

    a) Definition: delivery aided by device that provides traction or the means to rotate fetal head to occipitoanterior positions or to deliver head in breech presentations

    b) Types

        (1) Outlet forceps: Fetal skull has reached perineum, and scalp is visible between contractions, with sagittal suture no more than 45° from midline.

        (2) Low forceps: Fetal skull is at 2+ station or below.

        (3) Midforceps: Fetal skull is engaged, but presenting part of skull is above 2+ station.

c) Indications
    (1) Maternal: second-stage dystocia, exhaustion, when client's life is endangered
    (2) Fetal: distress, abnormal presentation, arrest in rotation
d) Prerequisites
    (1) Fully dilated cervix
    (2) Knowledge of exact position and station of fetal head
    (3) Ruptured membranes
    (4) Vertex or face presentation
    (5) No cephalopelvic disproportion
    (6) Regional anesthesia
e) Essential nursing care
    (1) Explain procedure and necessity to client and support person.
    (2) Encourage continuation of breathing techniques.
    (3) Continuously monitor maternal status as physician applies traction with each contraction.
    (4) Monitor fetal heart rate pattern (transient bradycardia with traction is common).
    (5) Reassure client and support person that fetal facial bruising and edema are transient.
    (6) Assess for vaginal or cervical lacerations after delivery.

3. Vacuum extraction
  a) Definition: delivery aided by vacuum cup that applies suction to fetal head
  b) Indications: prolonged second stage of labor, fetal distress, arrest in fetal rotation, maternal disease (PIH, abruptio placentae, heart disease)
  c) Essential nursing care: providing education and support; after delivery, evaluating newborn for signs of irritation at application site and reassuring client and support person that caput succedaneum will subside

1. Libby is admitted to the labor and delivery unit in active labor. She is dilated 4 cm. Within the next 2 hours, her contractions lessen in frequency and become weak and inefficient. These are signs of:
   a. Hypertonic labor.
   b. Hypotonic labor.
   c. Precipitous labor.
   d. Secondary dysfunctional labor.

2. Libby's physician orders oxytocin augmentation. The desired effect of oxytocin is:
   a. Contractions every 5 minutes, lasting 30–40 seconds.
   b. Contractions every 2–4 minutes, of 40- to 60-second duration.
   c. Contractions every 2 minutes, of 90-second duration or more.
   d. Contractions every 4–5 minutes, lasting 40–60 seconds.

3. The nurse identifies a client in the first stage of labor with an occipitoposterior position. The nurse should anticipate that the client will have:
   a. Increased urge to void.
   b. Nausea and vomiting.
   c. Frequent leg cramps.
   d. Intense back pain.

4. The nurse is caring for a client with prolonged labor. She has identified a nursing diagnosis of high risk for infection related to increased need for invasive assessments. In planning nursing care related to this diagnosis, the nurse should:
   a. Monitor urine ketones.
   b. Evaluate temperature at least every 2 hours.
   c. Offer cool washcloths on the forehead.
   d. Perform vaginal exams with clean gloves.

5. Mrs. Pape has failed to progress in her labor. While completing a vaginal exam, the nurse identifies large fontanels, wide suture lines, and a thin, identifiable cranium. The head is not engaged. The nurse strongly suspects:
   a. Cephalhematoma.
   b. Hydrocephalus.
   c. Hydramnios.
   d. Caput succedaneum.

6. Mrs. Jhirad is admitted to the labor unit. By the prenatal records, the nurse identifies Mrs. Jhirad as being at 38 weeks' gestation and expecting twins. She is in active labor with membranes ruptured. Twin A is cephalic at −1 station. The physician orders electronic fetal monitoring. To obtain the most accurate assessment data, which monitoring mode should be employed?
   a. An external electronic monitor on each twin
   b. An internal monitor on twin A
   c. An internal monitor on twin A and an external monitor on twin B
   d. An internal monitor on each twin

7. The nurse is caring for a client who is HIV-infected and in active labor. The monitoring method of choice should be:
   a. A fetoscope.
   b. An external monitor.
   c. An internal monitor.
   d. Fetal scalp sampling.

8. While monitoring fetal heart rate with a continuous electronic fetal monitor, the nurse notes the presence of transient fetal accelerations with fetal movement. The initial nursing action is to:
   a. Reposition the woman on the left side.
   b. Begin oxygen by mask.
   c. Call the physician.
   d. Continue to monitor fetal status.

9. The physician orders prostaglandin gel (2 mg) for a client prior to the induction of labor with oxytocin. The rationale for use of the gel is to:
   a. Soften and efface the cervix.
   b. Stimulate uterine contractions.
   c. Decrease cervical pain receptors.
   d. Prevent cervical lacerations.

10. Linda is 30 hours postdelivery following an emergency cesarean section for cephalopelvic disproportion. She is very tired and weak and has not seen her newborn son since delivery. When asked if she would like to see him, she replies, "No, not now. He'll just cry and keep me from resting. This entire experience has been a nightmare." The most appropriate nursing diagnosis based on these data would be:
    a. Self-esteem disturbance related to inability to experience a vaginal birth.
    b. High risk for altered parenting related to lack of early contact.
    c. Situational low self-esteem related to loss of control.
    d. Knowledge deficit related to lack of understanding of infant bonding.

11. Zoa is a 16-year-old cocaine-addicted primipara who is admitted to labor and delivery. The nurse caring for Zoa needs to be alert for the possibility of cocaine-induced:
    a. Anxiety.
    b. Hypotension.
    c. Leg cramps.
    d. Hypertension.

12. While assessing Anna, a primigravida who is in labor, the nurse identifies the fetal presentation as breech. An appropriate nursing diagnosis for a breech presentation is:
    a. High risk for infection related to fetal presentation.
    b. High risk for fetal distress related to increased risk of prolapsed cord.
    c. Anxiety related to abnormal fetal development.
    d. High risk for injury related to maternal hypoxia.

1. **Correct answer is b.** In hypotonic labor, contractions decrease in frequency and intensity, slowing the dilatation and fetal descent.

   a. Hypertonic labor is characterized by painful, uncoordinated contractions that do not cause cervical dilatation. This usually occurs in the latent stage of labor.
   c. Precipitous labor is defined as labor that lasts less than 3 hours from onset of contractions.
   d. Secondary dysfunctional labor is impaired bearing-down efforts that prevent normal progression of labor. This occurs during the second stage of labor.

2. **Correct answer is b.** The nurse should expect a desired effectiveness with oxytocin of contractions every 2–4 minutes of 40- to 60-second duration.

   a and d. Neither of these contraction patterns indicate effectiveness of the oxytocin.
   c. If contractions occur every 2 minutes with a 90-second duration, the nurse should recognize this as a potentially dangerous situation due to hyperstimulation of the uterus.

3. **Correct answer is d.** Pressure from the fetal head against the mother's sacrum causes intense back pain.

   a. There is little relationship between ROP and LOP positions and bladder pressure.
   b and c. Nausea and vomiting and leg cramps may occur throughout labor but do not relate to fetal position.

4. **Correct answer is b.** The nurse should monitor the client's temperature as an indication of possible infection.

   a. Urine ketones are done to evaluate maternal hydration status.
   c. Cool washcloths are comfort measures that are unrelated to infection.
   d. The nurse should use sterile gloves for vaginal checks.

5. **Correct answer is b.** Hydrocephalus is a fetal anomaly that causes dystocia. It is characterized by excessive accumulation of cerebral spinal fluid in the ventricles of the brain. This results in the enlargement of the cranium.

   a. A cephalhematoma is localized blood beneath the skull of a newborn due to a disruption of the vessels during birth.
   c. Hydramnios is excessive amounts of amniotic fluid.
   d. Caput succedaneum is localized edema on the fetal or newborn scalp, often associated with vacuum extractions.

6. **Correct answer is c.** During labor, it is necessary to monitor both twins. Since membranes have ruptured, twin A could have an internal monitor and twin B an external one to obtain the most accurate data.

   a. An external monitor could be used on each twin. However, since the membranes have ruptured, 1 twin could benefit from an internal monitor.
   b. Both twins need to be monitored.
   d. An internal monitor can be applied to only 1 twin.

7. **Correct answer is b.** The fetus of an HIV-infected woman needs to be monitored in the same respect as any other fetus. However, the choice of monitor should be an external one.

   a. A fetoscope is used for auscultation of fetal heart rate. However, for long-term monitoring during labor, an external monitor is more accurate.
   c. Internal monitoring requires the use of scalp electrodes that should not be used since this procedure may increase the infant's risk of exposure to HIV.
   d. Fetal scalp sampling should be avoided because it would increase the risk to the infant of exposure to HIV.

8. **Correct answer is d.** Transient fetal accelerations with fetal movement is a normal pattern and thus the nurse will continue to assess fetal heart status.

   a. There is no need to reposition the woman.
   b. Oxygen is not required at this time.
   c. It is not necessary to call the physician.

9. **Correct answer is a.** Prostaglandin gel is used to "ripen" the cervix prior to induction with oxytocin. Its use results in a higher success rate for inductions and a shorter induction time.

   b. Prostaglandin gel at this dosage does not usually stimulate uterine contractions. However, prostaglandin vaginal suppositories (20 mg) are used for induction in second-trimester abortions of intrauterine fetal demise.
   c. Prostaglandin gel does not decrease pain.
   d. Prostaglandin gel is not used to prevent cervical lacerations.

10. **Correct answer is b.** Since Linda has not yet spent time with her son and does not express a desire to do so, the nurse should identify high risk for altered parenting.

   a and c. The data presented do not support self-esteem disturbance or low self-esteem.
   d. Knowledge deficit is an inappropriate diagnosis at this time. It would not be a "teachable moment" since Linda is very tired.

11. Correct answer is d. Cocaine is a stimulant that increases the effect of norepinephrine. This leads to vasoconstriction and elevated pulse and respiratory rates. Cocaine-induced hypertension needs careful assessment from the nurse. Seizure precautions and neurologic assessments are required if hypertension is present.

a. Anxiety is present in all laboring women to some degree whether cocaine-dependent or not.
b. Hypotension is not an effect of cocaine use for reasons given in correct answer d.
c. Leg cramps often occur in the laboring woman and may or may not relate to cocaine abuse.

12. Correct answer is b. Breech presentations are always at risk of developing a prolapsed cord.

a. A breech presentation may prolong labor and thus create a risk for infection. The infection would not relate to fetal position but rather the time element between rupture of membranes and delivery of the child.
c. A breech presentation does not indicate fetal abnormalities.
d. The mother has no risk for hypoxia with a breech presentation.

9

Normal Newborn

NURSING HIGHLIGHTS

1. Complete assessments are necessary to determine how well the newborn adapts to extrauterine life and to detect problems.
2. Newborns need special nursing care to maintain a clear airway, maintain an adequate body temperature, prevent hemorrhage, and initiate feeding.
3. Parents need special nursing care to promote attachment to the newborn and acquire parenting skills and knowledge.
4. Although many aspects of newborn appearance are transient and spontaneously resolve with time, parents may need to be reassured.
5. The goal of infant feeding is to provide requirements to meet the nutritional and weight-gain needs of the newborn and the emotional and practical concerns of the family.

apnea—absence of spontaneous breathing

galactosemia—inherited autosomal recessive disorder of galactose metabolism, indicated by neonate's intolerance to milk

homocystinuria—inherited autosomal recessive disorder of homocystine metabolism

hypospadias—an abnormality of the penis in which the urethra opens on the underside

imperforate meatus—abnormally closed duct

maple syrup urine disease—an inherited metabolic disorder characterized by a maple syrup odor to the urine, vomiting, hypertonicity, and severe mental retardation

pathologic jaundice—abnormal condition in newborn that may occur within 24 hours of life; other indications include duration of more than 7–10 days or bilirubin increases of more than 5 mg/dl per day; resulting from accumulation of bilirubin in lipid tissue; may be caused by hemolytic disease

phenylketonuria (PKU)—an inherited metabolic disorder that can result in mental retardation if not treated with dietary modification

phimosis—constriction of the foreskin making it impossible to retract the foreskin

physiologic jaundice—condition in newborn that may occur in second or third day after birth; resulting from normal reduction in number of red blood cells; peaks at 3–6 days and disappears by tenth day

I. Adaptation of newborn to extrauterine life

See text pages
_____

A. Respiratory
    1. Factors involved in the initiation of breathing
        a) Physical: Strong contraction of diaphragm retracts the chest (negative intrathoracic pressure), forces out fluid from lungs, and stimulates inspiration.
        b) Sensory: Decreased ambient temperature after birth acts as a thermal stimulus.
        c) Chemical: Changes in blood, caused by transitory asphyxia during the birthing process, act as stimuli for breathing.
    2. Newborn respiratory characteristics
        a) Neonate should breathe within seconds of birth.
        b) Lung expansion may take several minutes to complete; initial respirations may be shallow and irregular.
        c) Normal respiration occurs along with periods of apnea, which may last 5–10 seconds.
        d) In first hours of birth, respiration is rapid during periods of intense activity.

e) Any obstruction causes respiratory distress and must be removed.

f) Chest and abdomen should rise with inspiration.

B. Cardiovascular

1. Foramen ovale, ductus arteriosus, and ductus venosus close, triggered by initiation of respiration.

2. Umbilical arteries and vein and hepatic arteries eventually become ligaments.

3. Increase in blood volume contributes to conversion of fetal circulation to neonatal circulation.

a) Arterial pressure rises with loss of placenta.

b) Size of increase of blood volume depends on when umbilical cord is clamped.

c) Increased oxygen stimulates vasodilatation.

d) Blood pressure (BP) varies due to changes in blood volume, and it will vary with activity. (See section II,B,1,c of this chapter for BP at rest.)

4. Heart rate at birth accelerates to 175–180 beats per minute (bpm), falls to 115 bpm at 4–6 hours, and levels at 120 bpm at 12–24 hours.

C. Hematologic

1. Hemoglobin initially declines due to decrease in neonatal red cell mass (physiologic anemia of infancy).

2. Leukocytosis occurs due to birth trauma.

3. Platelet count and aggregation ability are the same as in adults.

4. Hematologic values are affected by several factors.

a) Site of blood sample: Capillary blood has higher levels of hemoglobin and hematocrit as compared with venous blood; therefore, several venous sites should be sampled to assure accuracy.

b) Placental transfusion: Delayed cord clamping and normal shift of plasma to extravascular spaces cause higher levels of hemoglobin and hematocrit.

c) Gestational age: Increased gestational age is associated with increased numbers of red blood cells and hemoglobin.

d) Hemorrhage: Prenatal and/or perinatal hemorrhage decreases hematocrit levels and total blood volume and predisposes to hyperbilirubinemia.

D. Metabolic: temperature regulation

1. Factors influencing body temperature

a) Newborns are homeothermal; they attempt to maintain internal (core) temperature within narrow range despite significant external variations.

b) Newborns are predisposed to heat transfer; they have limited subcutaneous fat and large surface area in relation to body weight.
2. Mechanisms of heat loss in newborn
   a) Convection: loss to surrounding air
   b) Radiation: loss to cooler object not in direct contact with newborn
   c) Conduction: loss to cooler object in direct contact with newborn
   d) Evaporation: loss to air from moisture on skin or in lungs
3. Ways newborns conserve heat and increase heat production
   a) Increased basal metabolic rate
   b) Increased muscular activity, although shivering is rare
   c) Chemical reaction, fueled by newborn stores of brown adipose tissue
   d) Peripheral vasoconstriction
   e) Assumption of fetal position

E. Hepatic
   1. The liver stores enough iron to last through the first 5 months when diet is primarily milk and deficient in iron.
   2. The liver continues prenatal function of blood formation and coagulation factors.
   3. Physiologic jaundice occurs as a normal biologic response.
      a) Occurs after first 24 hours of life; peaks at 3–5 days in term infant and 5–6 days in preterm infant; bilirubin levels should not exceed 13 mg/dl in term infant or 15 mg/dl in preterm infant
      b) Caused by increased production of bilirubin from lysis of red blood cells, decreased clearance of bilirubin, hepatic immaturity, and increased absorption of bilirubin from intestinal tract
      c) Must be distinguished from pathologic jaundice, in which levels rise within 24 hours of life

F. Gastrointestinal
   1. Breathing, sucking, and swallowing reflexes necessary for feeding are coordinated at birth in term infant.
   2. First passage of meconium (waste substance formed in utero from amniotic fluid and constituents) occurs within 24 hours of birth; meconium stools are passed for first few days of life; stools change to greenish brown and then yellowish brown; they may contain milk curds; nature of subsequent stools is dependent on whether infant is breastfed or bottle-fed.
   3. Daily number of stools decreases from 5–6 to 1–2 by about 1 week; breastfed infant may have stools more frequently.
   4. Newborn is not able to move food from lips to pharynx; therefore, nipple must be placed well inside baby's mouth.
   5. Well-developed sucking pads are present in cheeks.
   6. Most enzymes are available at birth, allowing newborn to digest simple carbohydrates and protein; unavailability of amylase and lipase decreases newborn's ability to digest complex carbohydrates and fats.

G. Renal
 1. Most newborns void within 24 hours.
 2. Kidney function in newborns is not complete. Newborns' inability to fully concentrate urine and their low dilutional capability must be considered when monitoring effect of excessive insensible water loss or restricted fluid intake.
 3. Urine may initially appear cloudy due to high mucus and urate content.
 4. Red or pink diaper stains are caused by uric acid crystals in urine; may be confused with blood.
 5. After 2–3 days, newborn urinates 10–15 times daily.

H. Immunologic
 1. Immunoglobulin G (IgG) antibody: is passed from pregnant woman to fetus; results in passive acquired immunity; is active against bacterial toxins
    a) IgG is the only immunoglobulin to cross the placenta.
    b) IgG is transferred during third trimester, making preterm infants more susceptible to infection.
 2. IgM: is produced by fetus beginning at 10–15 weeks' gestation; increased levels indicate exposure to intrauterine infection
 3. IgA: is passed to newborn in colostrum (forerunner of breast milk); provides some passive immunity

I. Neurologic
 1. Nervous system is immature at birth; movements are uncoordinated.
 2. Behavioral characteristics of newborns are variations in state of consciousness, or sleep-wake cycles.
    a) Sleep states
       (1) Deep, or quiet, sleep: delayed responses to external stimuli
       (2) Active REM sleep: irregular respirations and movement; responsive to external stimuli
    b) Alert states: drowsy or semidozing, wide awake, active awake, and crying
    c) Newborn behavior capacities
       (1) Habituation: ability to process and respond to stimulation; response can be decreased after repeated stimulation
       (2) Orientation: ability to follow and fixate on visual stimuli
       (3) Consolability: ability to use own resources for comfort
    d) Newborn sensory capacities
       (1) Auditory: ability to respond to stimulation with definite behavior repertoire; especially responsive to maternal sounds
       (2) Olfactory: ability to select by smell

      (3) Taste: ability to distinguish different tastes; responds with sucking pattern variations

      (4) Touch: ability to receive and process tactile stimulation

  3. Reflexes (see also section II,B,17 of this chapter)

    a) Presence or absence of reflexes reflects degree of maturity of neurologic system; persistence or absence of expected reflexes may indicate abnormality, possibly due to influence of maternal analgesia or anesthesia.

    b) Reflexes are important for survival, to aid feeding, and to stimulate human interaction.

II. Assessment of the newborn

A. Initial newborn assessment: done in birthing area to determine whether newborn is stable enough to stay with parents or whether resuscitation or immediate interventions are necessary (see Nurse Alert, "Abnormal Newborn Breathing Patterns")

  1. Take Apgar score, a system used to evaluate infants at 1 and 5 minutes after birth; assesses 5 signs; scores for each sign are 0–2, with 2 being maximum; total score should be 8–10.

    a) Heart rate: Rate should be 150–180 bpm at 1 minute; slows to 130–140 bpm at 5 minutes; increases with crying; if absent or less than 100 bpm, resuscitation is needed.

See text pages
_____

! NURSE *ALERT* !

Abnormal Newborn Breathing Patterns

General signs
- Nasal flaring
- Chest retractions
- Grunting
- Use of accessory muscle
- Chin tug
- Labored breathing
- Cyanosis

Abnormal breath sounds
- Rhonchi
- Continued rales
- Wheezing
- Stridor
- Expiratory grunting

Abnormal respiratory rates
- Tachypnea: rate ≥60 breaths per minute
- Bradypnea: rate ≤25 breaths per minute

        b) Respiratory effort: Newborn should have no difficulty with breathing (normal respirations, 30–60 per minute); crying is vigorous; intercostal or xiphoid retraction, nasal flaring, cyanosis, and grunting are signs of respiratory depression.

        c) Muscle tone: Newborn should keep extremities flexed and resist extension.

        d) Reflex irritability: Slap on sole should provoke vigorous cry.

        e) Color: Body should become pink within 3 minutes of birth; even healthy infants may have bluish extremities for a short time.

2. Check overall appearance for anything unusual.
3. Examine head, face, front, back, and extremities for obvious defects or evidence of trauma.
4. Check nares for patency and for flaring. Remove mucus from nose and mouth, if present.
5. Examine skin for color and presence of staining or peeling.
6. Auscultate lungs for side-to-side comparison and efficiency of air exchange.
7. Take apical pulse.
8. Monitor temperature; prevent hypothermia.
9. Examine umbilical cord; it should have 2 arteries and 1 vein.
10. Palpate liver for enlargement.
11. Weigh neonate, and measure length and head circumference.
12. Make rapid estimate of gestational age; gestational age is 39 weeks or older if:
    a) Soles are covered with creases.
    b) Breast nodule diameter is 7 mm.
    c) Scalp hair is coarse and silky.
    d) Earlobes are stiffened by thick cartilage.
    e) In male, testes are pendulous, scrotum is full, rugae is extensive.
    f) In female, labia majora are large and cover clitoris and labia minora.
13. Be sure neonate has proper identification band.

B. Expanded physical assessment: done periodically during stay in hospital or birth center to evaluate neonate's progress in adapting to extrauterine life (see Nurse Alert, "Common Variations in the Newborn")

1. Vital signs
   a) Temperature: normal axillary range: 97.7°F–98.6°F; should be monitored every hour until stable, then every 8 hours
   b) Apical pulse
      (1) Pulse should be monitored every 15–30 minutes for first hour, then every 1–2 hours for 3 hours, and every 8 hours thereafter.

   (2) Variations in heart rate are normal: 100 bpm while asleep, 120–160 bpm while awake, 180 bpm while crying.

  c) Blood pressure: average BP at rest, 74/46 mm Hg; should be taken with Doppler device for accuracy; usually done only once unless abnormal

  d) Respirations: normal, 30–60 respirations per minute

  e) Weight at birth: 2700–4000 g; should be done at birth and daily at same time each day

   (1) Scales are covered to prevent spread of infection and heat loss from conduction.

   (2) Weight is correlated with determination of gestational age.

   (3) Weight is influenced by racial origin, maternal age, size of parents, maternal nutrition, and placental perfusion.

   (4) Neonate loses 5%–10% of birth weight in first 3–4 days.

  f) Measurements at birth

   (1) Length: 45–55 cm

   (2) Circumference of head: 33–37 cm

   (3) Circumference of chest: 31–35 cm

2. Expanded assessment of gestational age

  a) Purpose: to identify problems that may develop if newborn is preterm or has weight inappropriate for gestational age

  b) Components: evaluation of external physical characteristics and neurologic and/or neuromuscular developmental level; charts and scoring systems may be used

  c) Physical characteristics of full-term infant (see also section II,A,12 of this chapter)

   (1) Skin: parchment, deep cracking, absence of superficial blood vessels and vernix caseosa (white, pasty substance that protects skin of fetus)

   (2) Lanugo (fine body hair): almost absent, perhaps some on shoulders

      d) Neuromuscular maturity

        (1) Resting posture: Hypertonic flexion of all extremities is present in term newborns.

        (2) Recoil test: Extremities are extended; more complete and rapid recoil is accomplished by term newborns.

        (3) Square window sign: Hand is flexed toward ventral forearm; hand of term infant can be flexed onto the arm; larger angle is formed by premature newborn.

        (4) Popliteal angle: Thigh is bent to chest; lower half of leg is extended until resistance is met; resistance increases with stage of maturity.

        (5) Scarf sign: Arm is drawn across chest; higher degrees of resistance indicate older gestational age.

        (6) Heel-to-ear maneuver: Foot is moved toward ear on same side; higher degrees of resistance indicate older gestational age.

3. Laboratory determinations

    a) Blood glucose: >45 mg/dl

    b) Hematocrit: <65%–70% (central venous sample)

4. Pattern of behavior during first several hours after birth (periods of reactivity)

    a) First period of reactivity (lasts up to 30 minutes after birth): Newborn is awake and active, and sucking reflex is strong; this is ideal time to initiate breastfeeding.

    b) Sleep phase (lasts 2–4 hours): Bowel sounds appear; heart and respiratory rates decrease; newborn is difficult to arouse.

    c) Second period of reactivity (lasts 4–6 hours): Newborn is alert but may have apneic periods requiring stimulation; mucus increases and may cause choking or gagging; first meconium and urine are passed.

5. Skin: should be smooth; flexible, yet elastic; ruddy colored; warm to the touch

    a) Normal variations

      (1) Acrocyanosis: bluish discoloration of hands and feet; transient

      (2) Harlequin sign: blood vessels dilate on one side of the body and not the other; transient

      (3) Jaundice: yellowish color first detectable on face when bilirubin is >6 mg/dl; should subside within 3–5 days

      (4) Erythema toxicum: widespread rash; does not occur on palms or soles; no known cause or treatment; spontaneously disappears

(5) Milia: plugged sebaceous glands especially on nose; disappear spontaneously

b) Birthmarks

(1) Telangiectatic nevi (stork bites): pink spots on eyelids or nose; fade during infancy

(2) Mongolian spots: bluish-black areas on dorsum and buttocks; found commonly in Asian and dark-skinned infants; subside during infancy

(3) Nevus flammeus (port wine stain): dark-red capillary angioma; does not fade

(4) Nevus vasculosus (strawberry mark): dark-red capillary hemangioma; usually resolves by 7 years

6. Head: should be approximately 25% of body size

a) Variations in head shape, size, or appearance

(1) Craniostenosis: premature closure of cranial sutures; will require surgical intervention to avoid brain compression

(2) Molding: asymmetry due to overriding of cranial bones during labor and birth

(a) Molding diminishes and suture lines become palpable within a few days.

(b) Parents need reassurance that molding is transient.

(c) Newborns delivered in breech presentation or by cesarean section do not experience molding.

(3) Soft tissue edema and bruising

(a) Cephalhematoma: pocket of blood resulting from ruptured blood vessels between surface of cranial bone and periosteal membrane; common in vertex births; does not cross suture line; spontaneously resolves

(b) Caput succedaneum: pocket of serum under scalp; results from difficult labor or vacuum extraction; crosses suture line

b) Fontanels (junctures of cranial bones)

(1) Types

(a) Anterior: diamond-shaped; 3–4 cm long and 2–3 cm wide; closes by 18 months

(b) Posterior: triangular; smaller than the anterior; closes by 8–12 weeks (occasionally closed at birth)

(2) Normal variations: swell with crying, pulsate with heartbeat

(3) Abnormal deviations: bulge with increased intracranial pressure, become depressed with dehydration

7. Face: should be symmetrical when resting and crying; cheeks should be full

a) Variation: Paralysis can occur on one side from forceps delivery or compression of facial nerve during childbirth; usually resolves spontaneously.

      b) Eyes

         (1) Should be symmetrically placed; should have blink reflex and red reflex and ability to track objects to midline; pupils should be equal and reactive; some newborns have tears

         (2) Common variations that will disappear: chemical conjunctivitis resulting from instillation of ophthalmic drops, subconjunctival hemorrhage from increased ocular pressure at birth, transient strabismus

      c) Nose: should have midline placement, intact septum, patent nares, equal-size nostrils

      d) Ears: should be soft, pliable; cartilage should recoil easily; should have patent auditory canal

         (1) Placement: Top attachment of ear should be even with inner and outer canthi of eye.

         (2) Hearing: Infant should turn toward loud or moderate noises by 2 minutes.

      e) Mouth

         (1) Should have intact soft and hard palate; sucking pads inside cheeks; midline uvula; free-moving tongue; tongue proportional to mouth; gag, swallow, and sucking reflexes

         (2) Normal variations: Epstein's pearls (keratin-containing cysts that usually disappear in weeks), precocious teeth (may need to be extracted if loose)

   8. Neck: should be short, creased, move freely; neck control should be sufficient for infant to hold up head briefly; clavicles should be straight and intact

   9. Chest

      a) Should be round, symmetrical, 1–2 cm smaller than head

      b) Normal variations that will disappear: protruding xiphoid process (lower segment of the sternum); breast hypertrophy and secretion of milklike substance (so-called witch's milk), resulting from maternal hormone influences

      c) Breathing: Sounds are loud, bronchial, and equal bilaterally; movements are primarily diaphragmatic; breathing may be moist in first few hours, especially in newborn delivered by cesarean.

      d) Heart: regular rate and rhythm; distinct first and second heart sounds; possible presence of benign murmur in first few days (indicative of patent ductus arteriosus)

  10. Abdomen

      a) Should be cylindrical, protuberant without appearing distended; should have laxness of muscles

      b) Palpable liver, spleen, and kidneys

      c) Movements: synchronous with respirations

11. Umbilical cord: should have no extensive protrusion, bleeding, herniation, or signs of infection; should be dry and odorless; should have 2 arteries and 1 vein
12. Genitalia, female
    a) Labia majora, labia minora, and clitoris: should be appropriate size for gestational age
    b) Normal variations that will disappear: hymenal or vaginal tag; pseudomenstruation (vaginal discharge tinged with blood), resulting from withdrawal of maternal hormones
13. Genitalia, male
    a) Foreskin in uncircumcised boy: should cover glans (foreskin removed in circumcised boy)
    b) Urethral opening: should be at penile tip
    c) Testes: should be descended
    d) Scrotum: usually appears relatively large; if breech birth, may have edema and discoloration; should be inspected for hydrocele (collection of fluid around tissues)
14. Anus: should be patent and without fissure
15. Extremities: should be symmetrical and move through range of motion; should have proper number of digits
    a) Arms and hands: should be symmetrical and have normal palmar crease and normal movement
    b) Legs and feet: Legs should appear bowed; major gluteal folds should be even; there should be no "clunk" or "click" sound when leg is abducted; soles should be well lined or wrinkled; foot should align readily with manipulation.
16. Back
    a) Spine should be straight and flat and easily flexed.
    b) Infant can briefly raise head when prone.
17. Reflexes
    a) Tonic neck (fencer position): When head is turned to one side, extremity on same side straightens and on other side flexes; persists until third month.
    b) Grasping: When palm of hand is stimulated, fingers grasp (lessens at 3–4 months); when sole of foot is stimulated, toes curl under (lessens at 8 months).
    c) Moro: When infant is startled, arms and hands straighten outward and knees flex; arms then return to chest; fingers spread to form C; persists until 6 months.
    d) Rooting: When side of mouth is stroked, face turns toward that side.
    e) Sucking: When object is inserted in mouth or touched to lips, sucking follows.
    f) Babinski: When lateral aspect of sole is stroked upward and across ball of foot, toes hyperextend.

C. Assessment prior to discharge: done to evaluate readiness of client and infant for home care and to provide anticipatory guidance and teaching to parents
   1. Early discharge: Clients and newborns without complications are often offered option of leaving hospital within 24 hours of birth.
      a) Shortens period of observation and evaluation of newborn and instruction of parents
      b) Requires parents to take on responsibilities of postnatal care usually done at hospital
   2. Discharge teaching (same as section III,E of this chapter)

III. Essential nursing care

See text pages
_____

A. Nursing assessment
   1. Assess general characteristics, variations, and responses to determine need for further intervention (e.g., resuscitation).
   2. Evaluate airway clearance.
   3. Monitor temperature.
   4. Monitor respiratory rate, rhythm, and effort.
   5. Monitor heart rate and rhythm.
   6. Monitor skin color.
   7. Monitor activity level and muscle tone.
   8. Determine special needs of newborn.
   9. Determine special needs of family.

B. Nursing diagnoses
   1. Ineffective breathing pattern related to obstructed airway
   2. Ineffective thermoregulation (hypothermia) related to newborn status
   3. Potential for infection related to immature immune system
   4. High risk for injury related to maturational factors
   5. Altered nutrition, less than body requirements, related to parental knowledge deficit of newborn needs
   6. Altered nutrition, more than body requirements, related to parental knowledge deficit of newborn needs
   7. High risk for impaired skin integrity related to inadequate skin care
   8. Altered peripheral tissue perfusion related to hypothermia
   9. Altered patterns of bowel or urinary elimination related to inadequate fluid intake
   10. Parental knowledge deficit related to inexperience in infant care
   11. Altered family processes related to the need to integrate newborn into family unit

C. Nursing intervention
1. Have resuscitation equipment available and in good order.
2. Keep airway clear of mucus.
   a) Position newborn on side to aid in drainage.
   b) Use bulb syringe or mechanical suction device to remove mucus.
   c) Always keep bulb syringe near newborn.
   d) Teach parents how to use bulb syringe and how to care for choking infant.
3. Maintain thermoregulation.
   a) Wipe amniotic fluid from newborn's head and body as soon as possible.
   b) Use stockinette cap to prevent heat loss from head.
   c) Place thoroughly dried, unclothed newborn under radiant warmer (or in skin-to-skin contact with mother, then covered by 2 layers of material) until temperature stabilizes.
   d) Attach skin probe for ongoing monitoring of temperature.
   e) Provide temperature assessment.
      (1) Rectal: lubricated thermometer inserted ½ inch and held in place for 5 minutes (not recommended because of possible trauma; used only to check anal patency)
      (2) Axillary: thermometer held under arm for 3–4 minutes
4. Institute measures to control infection.
   a) Minimize exposure to organisms.
   b) Always wash hands before providing care.
   c) Do not allow ill personnel in delivery or nursery room.
   d) Monitor umbilical cord stump and circumcision site for signs of infection.
   e) Provide eye prophylaxis against gonorrhea and *Chlamydia* by instilling erythromycin ointment at birth.
5. Provide safe environment.
   a) Use firm grasp because newborns may be slippery.
   b) Ensure that area is warm, draft-free, well-lighted, and free of hazards.
   c) Check ID bands to match infant with mother.
   d) Monitor access to infants and mothers; limit to only those with appropriate ID.
6. Test for hypoglycemia: Use glucose test strip (Dextrostix) to estimate blood sugar levels upon admission to nursery; if <45 mg/dl, feed with 5%–10% glucose.
7. Bathe newborn.
   a) Delay bath until after body temperature stabilizes.
   b) Make sure room is warm and free of drafts.
   c) Bathe newborn quickly, exposing only one area at a time.
   d) Until first bath is complete, personnel must wear gloves when handling newborn (universal precautions for human immunodeficiency virus [HIV]).
   e) Proceed from "cleanest" to "most soiled" body areas.

8. Provide cord care.
   a) Use triple dye or antimicrobial agent such as bacitracin ointment.
   b) Remove cord clamp after 24 hours (cord should be dry).
   c) Cleanse base of cord daily with alcohol.
9. Dress newborn.
   a) Swaddling helps newborn maintain temperature, provides feeling of closeness, and often quiets fretting baby.
   b) Dress newborn in 1 more light layer than parent is wearing.
10. Prevent complications of hemorrhagic disease: administer prophylactic injection of vitamin K IM into vastus lateralis because newborn gastrointestinal tract is sterile and does not contain intestinal flora needed to synthesize vitamin K.
11. Provide care related to circumcision (surgical removal of foreskin to expose the glans).
    a) Check that consent form has been signed before procedure.
    b) Observe for signs of bleeding, drainage, or odor after circumcision.
    c) Keep area clean with soap and water or plain water; apply sterile petrolatum gauze after each diaper change.
    d) Fasten diapers loosely for 2–3 days.
12. Restrain newborn if necessary.
    a) Purposes
       (1) To facilitate examinations
       (2) To limit discomfort during tests, procedures, and collection of specimens
    b) Types of restraint
       (1) Mummy technique: used for more vigorous newborns and in tests that involve the head and neck
       (2) Extremity restraints: used to control movement of newborn's arms and legs; all 4 extremities must be restrained and padded with cotton
13. Handle and position newborn carefully: always support head and buttocks.
    a) Cradle hold is frequently used during feedings.
    b) Upright position provides security and a sense of closeness; it is also good for burping.
    c) Football hold allows eye contact with newborn and is a safe hold during ambulation with parent.
14. Promote and monitor adequate bowel elimination.
    a) Encourage early breastfeeding or bottle feeding; colostrum has laxative effect and will assist with meconium passage.
    b) Notify physician if meconium has not passed by 24 hours (sign of imperforate anus or gastrointestinal problems).

c) Record number, color, consistency of stools daily.

d) Report to physician watery or foul-smelling stools or those containing mucus.

15. Promote and monitor adequate urinary elimination.

a) Encourage early breastfeeding or bottle feeding.

b) Chart intake and output.

c) If newborn has not voided in 24 hours, notify physician (sign of imperforate meatus or renal problems).

16. Enhance parental knowledge.

a) Use a variety of opportunities to educate parents in care of newborn (e.g., encourage participation in routine care of newborn, such as feeding, bathing, and monitoring temperature); provide video or printed matter to reinforce retention.

b) Provide information on sleep, activity, and crying states.

(1) Individual variations are common, although for first several days most newborns sleep continuously when not feeding.

(2) In crying states, infant is uncomfortable, and cause needs to be identified.

(3) Parents will learn to distinguish tones and qualities of cries.

c) Enhance family interactions.

(1) Encourage parent-infant attachment as well as the involvement of other family members.

(2) Provide emotional support and encouragement, especially to new parents, regarding their competence in providing infant care.

D. Nursing evaluation

1. Newborn does not experience cardiopulmonary difficulties and establishes appropriate breathing pattern.

2. Temperature stabilizes and parents understand how to correctly evaluate the temperature of newborn.

3. Newborn does not show signs of umbilical cord infection and receives a bath and cord care.

4. Newborn receives prophylactic eye medication and does not develop eye problems.

5. Newborn receives prophylactic vitamin K and no hemorrhage occurs.

6. Newborn is circumcised if the parents wish; no infection or hemorrhage occurs.

7. Newborn has appropriate blood glucose level.

8. Bowel and bladder elimination are normal.

9. Parents learn how to care for their newborn and feel confident of their parenting capabilities.

10. Nurse recognizes problems early and institutes corrective measures; client and infant remain free of distress.

11. Newborn has made a successful adaptation to breastfeeding or bottle feeding.

12. Newborn has screening lab work done after 24 hours on breastfeeding or bottle feeding.

E. Discharge teaching
   1. Ensure that parents understand fundamentals of newborn care.
      a) Positioning and handling
      b) Normal newborn behavior
      c) Meeting needs for food and fluids (see also section IV,F of this chapter)
      d) Bathing
      e) Taking temperature
      f) Use of bulb syringe
      g) When to call physician (see Client Teaching Checklist, "Postdischarge Danger Signs")
   2. Provide information on safety.
      a) Infants should go home in car seat, which should always be used.
      b) Pillows and stuffed animals can cause suffocation.
      c) Crib should meet safety standards.
         (1) Slats no more than $2\frac{3}{8}$ inches apart
         (2) Snug-fitting mattress
   3. Provide information on newborn screening programs.
      a) Purpose: to detect disorders that cause mental retardation, physical handicaps, or death
      b) Examples: galactosemia, homocystinuria, hypothyroidism, maple syrup urine disease, phenylketonuria (PKU), sickle cell anemia
      c) Note: Infant needs to be on breastfeeding or bottle feeding at least 24 hours before newborn screening test will be valid.

✔ CLIENT TEACHING CHECKLIST ✔

Postdischarge Danger Signs

Instruct client to report these signs to a health care provider:

✔ Skin color changes: blue or yellow
✔ Temperature: >101°F or <96°F
✔ Vomiting: forceful or frequent
✔ Behavior: listless, hard to rouse, inconsolable crying or fussiness
✔ Apnea: cessation of breathing for >15 seconds
✔ Bleeding or abnormal discharge
✔ Changes in elimination: 2 or more green, watery stools; no wet diapers for 18–24 hours; or less than 6 wet diapers a day
✔ Refusal of 2 consecutive feedings
✔ Foul odor from cord or circumcision site (often first sign of infection)

---

4. Provide information on follow-up visits.
   a) Schedules and appointments
   b) Initial home visits if indicated
   c) Appropriate telephone numbers

IV. Newborn nutrition and feeding

See text pages

A. Nutritional needs
   1. Adequate carbohydrates, protein, fat, minerals, vitamins, and calories (50–55 cal/lb/day, 110–120 cal/kg/day)
   2. Adequate fluid: requirements are high because newborn cannot concentrate urine (64–73 ml/lb/day, 140–160 ml/kg/day)
   3. Weight gain
      a) First 6 months: 4–6 oz/week
      b) Second 6 months: 2–4 oz/week

B. Mechanisms of lactation
   1. Establishment of lactation occurs in 3 stages.
      a) Colostrum: thicker than breast milk, with more protein and minerals; rich in immunoglobulins; lasts for several days postpartum
      b) Transitional milk: high levels of fat, lactose, water-soluble vitamins, and calories; lasts for 2 weeks postpartum
      c) Mature milk: provides same caloric content as most formulas although it looks lighter; greater proportion of calories obtained from carbohydrates (lactose)
   2. Lactation is controlled by hormones, especially oxytocin and prolactin (from the pituitary gland).
      a) Oxytocin increases contractility of mammary ducts, causing milk secretion (let-down reflex).
      b) Prolactin promotes milk production.
      c) Let-down reflex is produced by stimulation of nerves in nipples as when newborn sucks, when mother hears the sound of a crying baby, or when mother thinks of children; reflex is inhibited by anxiety, stress, or discomfort.

C. Breastfeeding
   1. Advantages
      a) Immunologic
      b) Nonallergenic
      c) Nutritional
         (1) Aids digestion and absorption
         (2) Aids myelination and neurologic development
         (3) Aids metabolism of cholesterol
         (4) Provides high doses of minerals; iron supplementation not required for first 6 months
      d) Psychosocial
         (1) Enhances attachment and maternal-infant bond
         (2) Increases client's sense of accomplishment

   2. Disadvantages
      a) Drugs taken by mother are transmitted to infant through breast milk.
      b) Breast milk may cause transitory jaundice in about 1% of infants.
      c) Mother's poor nutrition, physical health, mental health, or work schedule may preclude breastfeeding.
   3. Contraindications
      a) Infant illness or infection (e.g., lactose-free diet required for infants with galactosemia)
      b) Maternal infection (e.g., HIV, cytomegalovirus, hepatitis B)
      c) Maternal medication (e.g., anticoagulants, oral contraceptives, psychotherapeutic drugs)

D. Bottle feeding
   1. Advantages
      a) May suit mores and pressures of socioeconomic class
      b) Allows mother to return to employment more easily
      c) Convenience, if using ready-to-feed formulas
      d) Encourages involvement of father and other family members in feeding
   2. Disadvantages
      a) Preparation time
      b) Sterilization concerns
      c) Possibility of infection
      d) Possibility of allergic reaction

E. Essentials of newborn feeding
   1. Initial feeding
      a) Determined by physiologic and behavioral cues
         (1) Active bowel sounds
         (2) Absence of abdominal distention
         (3) Lusty cry that quiets and is replaced by rooting and sucking behaviors when stimulus placed on lips
      b) Breastfeeding: can begin immediately after birth unless mother is heavily sedated, 5-minute Apgar score is less than 6, or infant is premature
      c) Bottle feeding: can begin at 1–4 hours after birth unless infant is unstable or premature
      d) Possible problems
         (1) Esophageal atresia: Feeding is taken well but contents are regurgitated unchanged.

(2) Tracheoesophageal fistula: Newborn gags, chokes, regurgitates mucus, and may become cyanotic.

(3) Cleft lip and/or cleft palate: Infant requires special nipple or modification with breastfeeding.

2. Establishing a feeding pattern
   a) For bottle-fed infants, every 3–4 hours on demand
   b) More often for breastfed infants because breast milk is digested faster than formula; also on demand

3. Promoting successful feeding
   a) Support maternal feeding-method decision.
   b) Facilitate the mother-infant bonding experience as much as possible.
   c) Provide client education.
   d) Refer to support group.

F. Parent education
1. Education for breastfeeding
   a) Self-demand schedule is usual practice.
   b) Mother should offer both breasts at each feeding for approximately 5–7 minutes per side; should alternate which breast is offered first at each feeding.
   c) Infant should be positioned with mouth toward nipple; ear, shoulder, and hip should be in direct alignment.
   d) Maternal position should vary with each feeding to empty breasts and prevent soreness.
   e) Mother must check to see that infant is sucking effectively, airway is not blocked, and swallowing is efficient.
   f) Infant is getting adequate intake if he/she is wetting 6–8 diapers daily, has at least 1 stool each day, is sleeping well, and is gaining weight steadily.
   g) Infant must latch on properly; areola should be almost completely covered by infant's mouth.
   h) Sucking behaviors vary.
   i) Mother should break suction between nipple and infant's mouth before attempting to remove infant from breast.
   j) Supplemental formula feeding is discouraged because it may lead to nipple confusion.

2. Special considerations in breastfeeding
   a) Clients with diabetes may need to decrease or readjust insulin dosage.
   b) Flexibility is possible: Milk can be expressed manually or with pump to allow others to feed the infant, to relieve breast fullness, and to help build up or maintain the milk supply.
   c) Decision of when to wean is individual and complex.
      (1) Process is easier if both mother and child are ready.
      (2) Process should be gradual: substitute one feeding from a cup or bottle for one breastfeeding session at a time.
   d) Breastfeeding problems benefit from anticipatory guidance (see Client Teaching Checklist, "Strategies for Relieving Common Breastfeeding Problems").

3. Education for bottle feeding
   a) Bottle should be held like pencil with nipple pointed directly into mouth; milk should fill nipple area so infant does not gulp air.
   b) Infant may be fed every 3–4 hours on demand.
   c) It is necessary to burp infant; it is normal for newborns to regurgitate frequently.
   d) In preparing formula, cleanliness is essential, but sterilization is necessary only if water supply is questionable.
   e) Nipples should be washed by hand.
   f) One day's supply can be prepared in advance.

✔ CLIENT TEACHING CHECKLIST ✔

Strategies for Relieving Common Breastfeeding Problems

Instruct client to do the following:

Nipple soreness
✔ Change nursing positions for each feeding.
✔ Start nursing on different breast for each feeding.
✔ Expose nipples to air.
✔ Avoid locally applied ointments; rub colostrum or breast milk onto nipple and areola after nursing.
✔ Limit sucking time; use pacifier if necessary.
✔ Wear breast pad to prevent irritation; avoid pads with plastic liners.
✔ Discontinue breastfeeding for 48 hours, manually expressing milk during this time.

Engorged breasts
✔ Increase frequency of feeding.
✔ Apply moist heat or stand in warm shower.
✔ Massage breast.
✔ Express milk manually or with a pump.
✔ Take mild analgesia 20 minutes before feeding, if discomfort is excessive.

Plugged ducts
✔ Before nursing, massage breasts during warm shower or after using warm compresses.
✔ Offer unaffected breast first.
✔ Nurse longer and more frequently.
✔ Change nursing positions.
✔ Use warm compresses after nursing.

4. Special considerations in bottle feeding
    a) There are 3 types of formulas: ready-to-feed, concentrate, and powder; parent must base selection on cost and convenience and must follow preparation directions for the type selected.
    b) Formula may cause lactose intolerance: Some infants cannot tolerate cow's milk and must be fed formulas made from substitutes such as soybeans.
    c) Formula is recommended for at least the first 6 months (preferably 1 year).

1. The nurse assesses Baby Boy A immediately after delivery. She notes that he has sole creases to his heels, coarse scalp hair, and extensive scrotal rugae. She estimates his gestational age as:
   a. 34 weeks.
   b. 36 weeks.
   c. 37–38 weeks.
   d. 39 weeks or more.

2. The best rationale for the immediate wiping of amniotic fluid and blood from the newborn's head and body is to:
   a. Facilitate ease of carrying the newborn.
   b. Minimize heat loss.
   c. Prevent transmission of blood-borne pathogens.
   d. Provide stimulation.

3. Newborns are given a single dose of 0.5–1 mg of phytonadione solution IM. This is done to prevent:
   a. Hyperbilirubinemia.
   b. Hypoprothrombinemia.
   c. Ophthalmia neonatorum.
   d. Hypoglycemia.

4. Apgar scores are routinely used for assessing the newborn at birth. The components of the Apgar system are:
   a. Heart rate, respiratory effort, muscle tone, and color.
   b. Heart rate, respiratory effort, muscle tone, and reflex irritability.
   c. Heart rate, respiratory effort, muscle tone, color, and temperature.
   d. Heart rate, respiratory effort, muscle tone, reflex irritability, and color.

5. Baby Girl S is given a 1-minute Apgar score of 3. This indicates a need for:
   a. Routine observations.
   b. Gentle rubbing and patting.
   c. Oxygen administration.
   d. Aggressive resuscitation.

6. Placental transfusion as a result of late cord clamping causes which of the following direct physiologic responses in the newborn?
   a. Leukocytosis
   b. Increased levels of hemoglobin and hematocrit
   c. Respiratory acidosis
   d. Higher renal threshold for glucose

7. Which of the following conditions would be abnormal during the first 12 hours of life?
   a. Heart rate 180 bpm while crying
   b. Blood glucose 50 mg/dl
   c. Protuberant abdomen
   d. Jaundice

8. Acrocyanosis is related to:
   a. Immature capillary function.
   b. Increased blood volume.
   c. Malfunctioning central nervous system (CNS).
   d. Apneic periods of the newborn.

9. Parents should be counseled to notify their health care provider when their newborn has:
   a. 2 or more green, watery stools.
   b. A temperature of 99.6°F.
   c. Periods of apnea lasting 10–15 seconds.
   d. A black, discolored umbilical cord.

10. The mother of Baby Girl S asks the nurse why she cannot give cereal to her newborn to help the baby sleep longer. The nurse's response is based on the understanding that:
    a. Newborns do not have amylase available to digest complex carbohydrates.
    b. A newborn's sleep cycle is only 3–4 hours at a time no matter what the infant eats.
    c. Newborns do not have the normal intestinal flora necessary to digest cereal.
    d. Newborns cannot swallow solid foods.

11. Mary is breastfeeding her newborn son. She asks the nurse, "How will I know if he is getting enough milk?" The best response by the nurse would be:

   a. "If he sleeps through the night, he is well-fed."
   b. "You won't know for sure until he is weighed at his 2-week checkup."
   c. "That's one disadvantage of breastfeeding—you never really know."
   d. "Your son will be getting enough milk if he is wetting 6–8 diapers daily and is sleeping well."

12. Monique tells the nurse that she has painful and sore nipples. After assessment, the nurse should instruct Monique to:

   a. Nurse only 1 breast for each feeding.
   b. Change nursing positions for each feeding.
   c. Discontinue breastfeeding.
   d. Apply moist heat to nipples.

ANSWERS

1. **Correct answer is d.** At 39 weeks or more, the newborn shows extensive scrotal rugae, coarse and silky scalp hair, and soles covered with creases. In addition, breast nodule diameter is 7 mm and the earlobe is stiff with thick cartilage.

   a and b. A newborn of 36 weeks or less has only anterior transverse sole crease; fine, fuzzy scalp hair; and very few scrotal rugae.
   c. A newborn 37–38 weeks old shows approximately two-thirds sole creases, fine and fuzzy hair, and an intermediate amount of scrotal rugae.

2. **Correct answer is b.** Newborns are very susceptible to heat loss. By drying the newborn as soon as possible, the nurse minimizes the heat loss due to vaporization.

Prevention of heat loss and cold stress promotes adequate oxygenation and controls apnea and acid-base balance.

   a. Indeed a newborn is less slippery and thus easier to handle after the amniotic fluid and blood are wiped away. However, this is not the primary rationale.
   c. Prevention of blood-borne pathogens is important. However, it is not the primary reason for the action.
   d. Stimulation of the infant does occur with the wiping of the skin. However, this is not the primary rationale.

3. **Correct answer is b.** A water-soluble form of vitamin K is given as a preventive measure against neonatal hemorrhage.

   a. Hyperbilirubinemia may result if a dose greater than 1 mg of vitamin K is given.
   c. Ophthalmia neonatorum is an eye infection in the newborn generally caused by gonococcal or chlamydial infections.
   d. Hypoglycemia is not treated with vitamin K.

4. **Correct answer is d.** The Apgar score has 5 components: heart rate, respiratory effort, muscle tone, reflex irritability, and color. Each of these is given a score of 0, 1, or 2, and then added for a total possible score of 10.

   a, b, and **c.** These are incorrect answers because they do not list the proper components.

5. **Correct answer is d.** An Apgar score of 3 requires immediate resuscitation. This is a newborn with obvious respiratory depression.

   a. Routine observations are appropriate for healthy newborns with Apgar scores of 7–10.
   b. Gentle rubbing and patting acts as an additional stimulus and is appropriate for newborns with Apgar scores of 4–6.
   c. Oxygen administration is appropriate for infants with Apgar scores of 4–6.

6. **Correct answer is b.** A delay in cord clamping results in an explosion of blood volume. This can cause increased levels of hemoglobin and hematocrit. It is important to remember that these levels can also be a result of the normal shift of plasma to extravascular spaces.

   a. Leukocytosis of 18,000/mm³ is normal at birth and decreases rapidly. This does not relate to late cord clamping.
   c. Respiratory acidosis is not a direct result of late cord clamping.
   d. It is normal for all newborns to have a higher renal threshold for glucose. This does not relate to late cord clamping.

7. **Correct answer is d.** Jaundice that occurs within 24 hours of life is considered pathologic.

   a. Heart rate of 180 bpm when crying is normal. Likewise, 100 bpm while sleeping is normal.
   b. Blood glucose of >45 mg/dl is normal.
   c. A protuberant abdomen is normal in the newborn.

8. **Correct answer is a.** Acrocyanosis, or bluish discoloration of hands and feet, is transient and reflects newborn's immature capillary function.

   b. An increased blood volume does not relate to acrocyanosis.
   c. Malfunctioning of the CNS would not be reflective of acrocyanosis.
   d. Acrocyanosis does not relate to apneic periods.

9. **Correct answer is a.** Two or more green, watery stools are not normal and may indicate a gastrointestinal problem.

   b. A temperature of 99.6°F is within normal range.
   c. Periods of apnea <15 seconds are normal.
   d. A black, discolored umbilical cord is part of the normal disintegration of the cord before it drops off.

10. **Correct answer is a.** Infants do not have amylase available to break down a complex carbohydrate such as cereal. Salivary amylase is not produced until 3 months of age.

    b. The newborn sleeps an average of 17 hours a day, waking for feedings and other comfort measures. However, this is not the reason why diluted cereal is inappropriate for the newborn.
    c. It is true that newborns are born with a sterile GI tract. However, soon after birth, oral and anal orifices allow bacteria in, thus establishing a normal flora.
    d. Newborns can swallow solid foods, although their efforts are uncoordinated.

11. **Correct answer is d.** Indicators for adequate intake are 6–8 wet diapers a day, at least 1 stool daily, weight gain, and adequate sleep.

    a. This is an inappropriate response because most newborns do not sleep through the night and this may or may not indicate adequate nutrition.
    b and **c.** These are incorrect for reasons stated in correct answer d.

12. **Correct answer is b.** Sore nipples may be prevented or limited by changing the nursing position for each feeding, as well as by using a correct position.

    a. When breastfeeding, it is important to use both breasts for each feeding. Alternating breasts for the start of each feeding may reduce nipple soreness.
    c. There is no need to discontinue breastfeeding.
    d. Moist heat should not be applied to sore nipples. Rather, the nipple should be exposed to the air. Use of a blow dryer or heat lamp after feedings can be beneficial.

10

High-Risk Conditions and Complications of the Newborn

NURSING HIGHLIGHTS

1. Early identification of at-risk newborns aids the nurse in making prompt diagnoses.
2. Neonatal problems must be corrected or minimized quickly to prevent permanent disability.
3. Many neonatal problems are similar although they may have different physiologic processes.
4. Nurse must understand normal physiology as well as abnormal conditions in the newborn in order to accurately observe responses to therapy and the development of complications.
5. Nurse is a primary source of information and emotional support for parents, who often require extra time and attention.
6. Support of grieving parents is an integral part of nursing responsibilities.

GLOSSARY

atelectasis—incomplete expansion or collapse of a lung

bilirubin—reddish-yellow bile pigment formed by breakdown of hemoglobin in red blood cells; water-insoluble, unconjugated form travels to liver, where it is converted to water-soluble, conjugated form and excreted in the bile

brown fat—specialized fat stores unique to the full-term neonate; utilized to generate heat

cold stress—hypothermia resulting in increased respirations and metabolic rate to maintain body temperature

Coombs' test—test for presence of antibodies that damage red blood cells; may be used to detect hemolytic disease in newborn

decerebrate posturing—position in which arms and legs are stiffly extended

hepatosplenomegaly—enlargement of liver and spleen

hypoglycemia—decreased blood glucose level, a common finding in the neonate, particularly after a stressful labor and/or delivery

lymphadenopathy—disorder of lymph nodes and vessels

opisthotonos—spasm causing back to arch acutely and head to bend back on neck

parotitis—inflammation of parotid salivary glands

phototherapy—exposure of newborn to intense fluorescent light; treatment for hyperbilirubinemia

polycythemia—abnormal increase in red blood cell volume

surfactant—substance that contributes to elastic properties of the lungs; lubricates lungs and decreases tendency of alveoli to collapse

ENHANCED OUTLINE

See text pages

I. Acquired disorders

A. Infants of mothers with diabetes mellitus
1. Risk factors: maternal type I diabetes (insulin-dependent) and maternal gestational diabetes (pregnancy-induced)
    a) Type I diabetes: Good maternal diabetic control during critical period of fetal organ development reduces congenital abnormalities.
    b) Gestational diabetes: Risk of infant mortality and morbidity and other complications is increased because maternal condition is not diagnosed until fetal organ development.

2. Complications
   a) Hypoglycemia: Maternal hyperglycemia results in fetal hyperglycemia; after delivery, newborn no longer receives maternal glucose, resulting in hypoglycemic state.
   b) Large-for-gestational-age infant: Increased insulin levels stimulate fetal organ growth, leading to increased organ size and macrosomia (large body size and weight).
   c) Hypocalcemia: Maternal hyperparathyroidism causes increase in serum calcium during pregnancy; after delivery, fetal serum calcium levels fall, resulting in hypocalcemia.
   d) Hyperbilirubinemia (same as section I,E of this chapter)
   e) Birth trauma, secondary to macrosomia
   f) Respiratory distress syndrome: High insulin levels can inhibit fetal lung maturation.
   g) Congenital abnormalities (heart, central nervous system, skeleton)
   h) Polycythemia: Condition is caused by decreased extracellular fluid volume and subsequent hemoconcentration.
   i) Small-for-gestational-age infant: In advanced diabetes, maternal vascular changes reduce effectiveness of placental perfusion, causing intrauterine growth retardation.
3. Essential nursing care
   a) Nursing assessment
      (1) Review client's health and obstetric record for history of diabetes to identify newborns at risk.
      (2) Observe newborn's physical condition for signs of complications associated with maternal diabetes.
      (3) Assess blood glucose level on admission; be prepared to start early feedings and/or administer intravenous (IV) glucose as ordered by physician.
   b) Nursing diagnoses
      (1) Altered nutrition, less than body requirements, related to increased glucose metabolism
      (2) Potential for injury related to macrosomia
      (3) High risk for impaired gas exchange related to respiratory distress
      (4) Ineffective family coping related to illness of newborn
   c) Nursing intervention
      (1) Identify newborns at risk.
      (2) Make preparations to resuscitate newborn with respiratory distress syndrome and to treat birth trauma resulting from large size.
      (3) Intervene for metabolic problems (e.g., hypoglycemia or hypocalcemia [see Nurse Alert, "Signs of Neonatal Hypoglycemia"]).
      (4) Monitor blood glucose levels frequently to evaluate effectiveness of early feedings and/or IV glucose.
      (5) Monitor lab tests (e.g., hematocrit) as needed.

      d) Nursing evaluation
        (1) Problems related to respiratory distress and altered metabolism are minimized.
        (2) Birth injuries are treated promptly.
        (3) Parents verbalize concerns about newborn's health problems.

B. Infection (sepsis neonatorum)
  1. Modes of transmission: in utero, during delivery, during resuscitation, or in the nursery (nosocomial infection)
  2. Types
    a) Bacterial infections: gastroenteritis, staphylococcal infections (most skin infections, a type of pneumonia), syphilis, conjunctivitis, thrush, navel infections, group B streptococci
    b) TORCH infections: *t*oxoplasmosis, *r*ubella, *c*ytomegalovirus, *h*erpes simplex virus (*O* may stand for *o*ther infections [e.g., hepatitis B])
  3. Risk factors
    a) Maternal: smoking; low socioeconomic status; minority race; bacterial or viral infection of the urinary tract, vagina, or cervix at delivery; premature rupture of membranes; prolonged second stage of labor
    b) Fetal/neonatal: prematurity, congenital abnormality, invasive procedure

---

!   N U R S E *A L E R T*   !

Signs of Neonatal Hypoglycemia

- Lethargy
- Jitteriness
- Vomiting
- Poor feeding
- High-pitched cry
- Difficult respirations
- Pallor
- Glucose test strip result ≤40 mg/dl assessed by Dextrostix or Accu-Check (requires immediate intervention) (Some clinicians use 45 mg as the cutoff for intervention.)

NOTE: Persistent abnormal levels of glucose indicated by Dextrostix or Accu-Check should be confirmed by laboratory analysis.

---

4. Complications: stillbirth, intrauterine infection, congenital malformation, chronic infection, meningitis, septic shock, infant death
5. Essential nursing care
    a) Nursing assessment
        (1) Review prenatal record and perinatal events for risk factors associated with infection.
        (2) Observe for signs of sepsis (see Nurse Alert, "Signs of Sepsis").
    b) Nursing diagnoses
        (1) High risk for infection related to immature immunologic system, environmental factors, maternal exposure, and sharing nursery
        (2) Impaired tissue integrity related to multiple invasive measures
        (3) Ineffective family coping related to present illness and prolonged hospital stay
    c) Nursing intervention
        (1) Prevent the spread of infection.
            (a) Promote strict policy of hand washing.
            (b) Clean and change all equipment at appropriate intervals.
        (2) Obtain cultures before administering antibiotics.
        (3) Administer antibiotics as ordered.
        (4) Promote well-being of newborn.
            (a) Provide respiratory, cardiovascular, nutritional, and fluid support.
            (b) Observe for metabolic and electrolyte disturbances.
            (c) Observe for response to treatment.
        (5) Provide emotional support and information to parents.
    d) Nursing evaluation
        (1) Risk factors associated with developing sepsis are identified early, and immediate intervention is instituted.
        (2) Appropriate aseptic techniques are used to prevent the spread of infection.

! NURSE ALERT !

Signs of Sepsis

- Subtle behavioral changes (lethargy and hypotonicity)
- Color changes (pallor, cyanosis, duskiness)
- Cool and clammy skin
- Temperature instability
- Poor feeding
- Hyperbilirubinemia
- Apnea

(3) Infection is effectively treated by antibiotics.

(4) Parents verbalize their concerns.

C. Acquired immunodeficiency syndrome (AIDS): an infectious disease caused by the human immunodeficiency virus (HIV) that compromises the immune system

1. Modes of transmission: transplacental, in breast milk, during infusion of contaminated blood

2. Diagnosis: enzyme-linked immunosorbent assay (ELISA); Western blot to detect HIV antibodies; evidence of immunosuppression, wasting syndrome, encephalopathy, and opportunistic disease to confirm diagnosis

   a) Newborns less than 6 months old may show false-positive test results due to the presence of maternal antibodies.

   b) Such newborns should be serially tested.

3. Risk factors: maternal history of IV drug abuse or needle sharing and sexual partner who tests positive for HIV antibodies

4. Complications

   a) Congenital abnormalities, especially neurologic

   b) Opportunistic infections

   c) Central nervous system dysfunction

   d) Facial abnormalities

5. Essential nursing care

   a) Nursing assessment

      (1) Observe newborn for signs of prematurity, intrauterine growth retardation, and failure to thrive.

      (2) Observe newborn for signs of opportunistic infection such as oral candidiasis (thrush) and chronic diarrhea.

      (3) Assess newborn for presence of generalized lymphadenopathy, hepatosplenomegaly, and parotitis.

   b) Nursing diagnoses

      (1) High risk for infection related to immunosuppression

      (2) Altered nutrition, less than body requirements, related to formula intolerance and inadequate intake

      (3) High risk for altered growth and development related to lack of attachment and stimulation

      (4) High risk for ineffective family coping related to AIDS diagnosis

   c) Nursing intervention

      (1) Continue to observe for signs of infection.

      (2) Monitor fluid intake and output and stool loss.

      (3) Provide frequent, small feedings.

      (4) Encourage family members to express their concerns and to participate in caretaking activities.

d) Nursing evaluation
  (1) Incidence of infection is minimized.
  (2) Newborn gains weight and follows normal growth curve.
  (3) Family members verbalize fears and begin to bond with infant.

D. Infants of substance abusers
  1. Risk factor: maternal abuse of alcohol and drugs during pregnancy
  2. Complications
    a) Fetal alcohol syndrome (FAS)
      (1) Growth retardation
      (2) Mental retardation
      (3) Feeding difficulties
      (4) Central nervous system problems
      (5) Distinctive facial abnormalities
    b) Substance withdrawal in newborn (see Nurse Alert, "Signs of Drug Withdrawal in Newborn")
    c) Intrauterine asphyxia resulting from fetal withdrawal secondary to maternal withdrawal
    d) Low birth weight
    e) Poor Apgar scores
    f) Respiratory distress
    g) Neglect related to continued maternal drug dependence
  3. Essential nursing care
    a) Nursing assessment
      (1) Review prenatal record for history of alcohol or drug abuse and last known intake.
      (2) Review obstetric events for delivery complications.
      (3) Observe newborn for evidence of behavioral and congenital abnormalities.

! NURSE *ALERT* !

Signs of Drug Withdrawal in Newborn

- Hyperactivity
- Jitteriness
- Irritability
- High-pitched cry
- Vomiting
- Diarrhea
- Stuffy nose
- Abnormal sleep-wake cycle (inability to sleep)
- Frequent sneezing and yawning
- Hypertonicity
- Poor sucking

> (4) Observe newborn for signs and symptoms of withdrawal within 6–12 hours and for at least 3 days.
>
> (5) Obtain blood for drug screen in suspected cases.

b) Nursing diagnoses

> (1) Altered nutrition, less than body requirements, related to uncoordinated sucking and swallowing
>
> (2) High risk for fluid volume deficit related to vomiting and diarrhea
>
> (3) Altered growth and development related to effects of maternal substance abuse
>
> (4) Altered parenting related to newborn's hyperirritable condition and potential continuation of maternal drug abuse

c) Nursing intervention

> (1) Provide newborn with nutritional and fluid support; supplement small, frequent feedings parenterally if necessary.
>
> (2) Administer medications as ordered for controlling withdrawal symptoms and weaning from substance.
>
> (3) Decrease environmental stimulation and swaddle newborn to decrease irritability.
>
> (4) Provide emotional support to parents and refer them to community resources for assistance and treatment.
>
> (5) Collaborate with other health care providers to determine if referral to child protective services is needed (to ensure that infant is discharged to a safe environment).

d) Nursing evaluation

> (1) Newborn tolerates feedings, gains weight, and has normal number of stools.
>
> (2) Newborn demonstrates less irritability and muscle rigidity.
>
> (3) Parents verbalize concerns and understand how to use community resources.

E. Neonatal jaundice (hyperbilirubinemia): accumulation of bilirubin in lipid tissue that results in yellow discoloration of skin

1. Types

   a) Physiologic jaundice: normal phenomenon

   b) Pathologic jaundice: variety of causes

   > (1) Hemolytic disease of the newborn secondary to Rh or ABO incompatibility
   >
   > (2) Increased production or decreased excretion of bilirubin

2. Risk factors: fetal or neonatal asphyxia, hypothermia, hypoglycemia, infection, polycythemia, excessive dose of vitamin K

3. Complications: kernicterus (buildup of bilirubin in brain cells, leading to spasticity, deafness, and mental retardation) and infant death

4. Essential nursing care
   a) Nursing assessment
      (1) Identify prenatal and perinatal risk factors for jaundice.
      (2) Observe for signs of jaundice within first 24 hours.
      (3) Monitor results of diagnostic tests (e.g., direct Coombs' test and maternal-neonatal blood typing).
   b) Nursing diagnoses
      (1) High risk for injury (neurologic) related to:
          (a) Elevated bilirubin level
          (b) Phototherapy
      (2) High risk for fluid volume deficit related to effects of phototherapy
      (3) High risk for injury related to exchange transfusion rebound
      (4) Anxiety (parental) related to diagnosis and need for phototherapy
   c) Nursing intervention
      (1) Monitor bilirubin level.
      (2) Give frequent feedings to encourage elimination of conjugated bilirubin in stool.
      (3) Initiate phototherapy as ordered: remove newborn's clothing, apply protective shields to eyes and male genitalia, monitor temperature of infant and isolette, monitor hydration status, and reposition newborn frequently.
      (4) Observe for diarrhea; thoroughly clean perineal area.
      (5) Prepare and assist with exchange transfusion.
      (6) Monitor for effects of exchange transfusion rebound: hyperbilirubinemia, electrolyte imbalance, hypoglycemia, hypothermia.
      (7) Provide parents with information about treatment of hyperbilirubinemia.
   d) Nursing evaluation
      (1) Newborn at risk for jaundice is promptly identified.
      (2) Newborn tolerates feedings and remains well hydrated.
      (3) Newborn's eyes and genitalia (male) are protected, and appropriate temperature and hydration status are maintained during phototherapy.

II. Gestational age and birthweight disorders

See text pages

A. Small-for-gestational-age (SGA) newborn
   1. Definition: newborn delivered at term who weighs less than 2500 g (below the tenth percentile for weight); condition referred to as intrauterine growth retardation (IUGR)
   2. Types
      a) Symmetric: caused by long-term maternal conditions or fetal genetic abnormalities; results in chronic prolonged retardation of growth that is proportional

      b) Asymmetric: caused by acute compromise of uteroplacental blood flow; birth weight disproportional to head size

3. Risk factors

      a) Maternal: malnutrition; vascular complications (e.g., pregnancy-induced hypertension); preexisting disease (e.g., diabetes and cardiac dysfunction); smoking; exposure to x-rays; substance abuse; placental conditions (e.g., placenta previa); lack of prenatal care

      b) Fetal: congenital infections, congenital abnormalities, multiple gestation

4. Complications: asphyxia, meconium aspiration syndrome, difficulty maintaining thermal regulation, hypoglycemia, hypocalcemia, polycythemia, learning disabilities, neurologic problems

5. Essential nursing care

      a) Nursing assessment

         (1) Identify risk factors for IUGR.

         (2) Examine newborn for signs of IUGR (see Nurse Alert, "Characteristics of Newborn with Intrauterine Growth Retardation").

         (3) Perform gestational age assessment.

         (4) Obtain lab work, including blood glucose, hematocrit, bilirubin, and calcium levels.

      b) Nursing diagnoses

         (1) Impaired gas exchange related to meconium aspiration

         (2) Hypothermia related to decreased subcutaneous fat (cold stress)

         (3) Altered tissue perfusion related to increased blood viscosity

         (4) High risk for altered parenting related to prolonged separation of newborn and parents

         (5) Knowledge deficit (parental) related to care of SGA newborn at home

      c) Nursing intervention

         (1) Prepare for possible resuscitation, auscultate breath sounds, and suction airways as needed.

         (2) Observe for signs of worsening respiratory distress and report immediately.

         (3) Provide neutral thermal environment; monitor temperature continuously.

         (4) Initiate early feedings or IV glucose if necessary as ordered by physician to prevent or treat hypoglycemia.

         (5) Monitor blood glucose levels frequently to evaluate effectiveness of early feedings and/or IV glucose.

         (6) Educate parents on caring for newborn.

      d) Nursing evaluation

         (1) Newborn maintains spontaneous, unassisted, and regular respirations.

         (2) Newborn maintains body temperature.

         (3) Newborn's hemoglobin and hematocrit levels are within normal range.

         (4) Parents bond with newborn in the hospital and are prepared to care for the infant after discharge.

B. Large-for-gestational-age (LGA) newborn

  1. Definition: Newborn delivered at term who weighs more than 4000 g (above the 90th percentile for weight)

  2. Risk factors: maternal diabetes, genetic predisposition, male sex, multiparity

  3. Complications

    a) Birth trauma secondary to cephalopelvic disproportion

       (1) Soft tissue injuries: caput succedaneum, cephalhematoma, subconjunctival and retinal hemorrhages, ecchymoses, abrasions

       (2) Skeletal injuries: skull fracture and clavicle fracture

       (3) Nervous system injuries: arm paralysis and facial paralysis

    b) Higher rate of cesarean sections and oxytocin-induced births

    c) Hypoglycemia, hypocalcemia, and polycythemia

  4. Essential nursing care

    a) Nursing assessment

       (1) Review diabetic client's health and obstetric records.

       (2) Identify LGA newborn (perinatal history, ultrasound determinations, gestational age testing).

       (3) Check for complications: monitor vital signs; monitor laboratory tests for hypoglycemia, hypocalcemia, and polycythemia; observe for signs of birth trauma.

    b) Nursing diagnoses

       (1) Potential for impaired physical mobility related to birth injury

(2) Altered nutrition, less than body requirements, related to increased glucose metabolism

(3) Knowledge deficit (parental) related to birth injury, its cause, management and therapy, and prognosis

c) Nursing intervention

(1) Conduct intermittent assessments (evidence of birth-related injuries may not appear at initial assessment).

(2) Observe for metabolic problems; monitor blood glucose concentration.

(3) Initiate early feedings or IV glucose as ordered by physician to prevent or treat hypoglycemia.

(4) Carry out treatment orders for birth injury, hypoglycemia, and polycythemia, as necessary.

(5) Monitor blood glucose levels frequently to evaluate effectiveness of early feedings and/or IV glucose.

(6) Educate and reassure parents about the injury and about weight patterns to expect.

(7) Encourage parents to verbalize feelings and provide emotional support.

d) Nursing evaluation

(1) At-risk newborn is identified prior to delivery.

(2) Birth injuries are identified and managed promptly.

(3) Problems related to altered metabolism are minimized.

(4) Parents are knowledgeable about birth injury and its consequences, are able to express their emotions, and feel supported.

C. Postterm newborn

1. Definition: newborn delivered after completion of 42 weeks' gestation

2. Risk factors: primiparity, high multiparity (5 or more pregnancies), history of postterm pregnancies

3. Complications (postmaturity syndrome): cephalopelvic disproportion, shoulder dystocia, placental insufficiency leading to hypoglycemia and asphyxia, meconium aspiration, polycythemia, congenital abnormalities, seizures, cold stress

4. Essential nursing care

a) Nursing assessment

(1) Identify at-risk fetus by reviewing prenatal chart and determining gestational age.

(2) Examine newborn for signs consistent with a postterm newborn (see Nurse Alert, "Signs of Postterm Newborn").

      b) Nursing diagnoses
- (1) Hypothermia related to decreased liver glycogen and brown fat stores
- (2) Altered nutrition, less than body requirements, related to increased use of glucose
- (3) High risk for impaired gas exchange related to meconium aspiration
- (4) Potential for impaired physical mobility related to birth injury

      c) Nursing intervention
- (1) Prepare to resuscitate asphyxiated newborn at delivery.
- (2) Provide warm environment to counteract newborn's poor response to cold and decreased brown fat stores and liver glycogen levels.
- (3) Frequently monitor glucose and institute early feedings and/or IV glucose as ordered by physician.
- (4) Observe for signs of respiratory distress and report immediately.

      d) Nursing evaluation
- (1) Respirations are spontaneous, unassisted, and regular.
- (2) Newborn maintains normal body temperature.
- (3) Nutritional intake is adequate, reflected by normal blood glucose levels and expected weight gain.
- (4) Birth injuries are identified and managed promptly.

D. Preterm newborn
1. Definition: newborn delivered before 38 weeks' gestation
2. Risk factors:
    a) Maternal: disease, reproductive tract abnormalities, smoking, underweight, age extremes, history of preterm labor, pregnancy-induced hypertension, urinary tract or vaginal infection, premature rupture of membranes, chorioamnionitis, polyhydramnios, lack of prenatal care
    b) Fetal: anomalies, infection, multiple gestation

3. Pulmonary complications
   a) Respiratory distress syndrome (previously known as hyaline membrane disease)
      (1) Cause: insufficient production of surfactant
      (2) Result: alveolar collapse, diminished lung compliance, and atelectasis
      (3) Diagnosis: arterial blood gas showing hypoxia, hypercapnia, and respiratory or metabolic acidosis
      (4) Medical management: administration of oxygen and mechanical ventilation
      (5) Essential nursing care
         (a) Nursing assessment
            i)   Identify at-risk newborns: perform gestational age assessment, check prenatal and neonatal history, determine familial tendency, and check Apgar scores.
            ii) Perform physical examination to check for signs of respiratory distress; report immediately (see Nurse Alert, "Signs of Respiratory Distress").
            iii) Continuously measure oxygen-saturation levels.
         (b) Nursing diagnoses
            i)   Impaired gas exchange related to inadequate lung surfactant
            ii) Ineffective airway clearance related to increased secretions
            iii) High risk for altered nutrition, less than body requirements, related to inability to suck and swallow effectively
            iv) High risk for infection related to invasive procedures and inadequate immunologic response
            v)   High risk for altered parenting related to need for specialized care in neonatal intensive care unit
         (c) Nursing intervention
            i)   Monitor respiratory status by physical assessment and measurements of oxygen saturation and blood gases.
            ii) Administer humidified oxygen and medication as ordered.
            iii) Anticipate possible use of artificial surfactant, and monitor respiratory response.
            iv) Wean from ventilation support as improvement warrants to decrease risk for retinopathy of prematurity (see section II,D,8 of this chapter).
            v)   Institute resuscitation if apnea develops.

       vi) Provide adequate calories (see section II,D,7,d of this chapter for methods of feeding).

      vii) Observe for signs of infection; ensure that infection control measures are practiced, especially with ventilation equipment.

     viii) Provide information to parents about the special problems and needs of their preterm infant.

      ix) Provide emotional support to parents.

  (d) Nursing evaluation

       i) Newborn maintains respiration rate without apnea.

      ii) Newborn gains weight.

     iii) No signs of infection are detected.

     iv) Parents understand the special problems and needs of their preterm infant and are gradually able to participate in care.

b) Bronchopulmonary dysplasia: chronic lung disorder

  (1) Cause: Following mechanical ventilation, newborn remains dependent on oxygen and ventilator therapy.

  (2) Result: diminished lung compliance and tendency for atelectasis

  (3) Diagnosis: respiratory distress, oxygen dependence, rales, carbon dioxide retention

  (4) Medical management

    (a) Repeat efforts to wean from ventilation.

    (b) Prevent infection.

  (5) Essential nursing care

    (a) Nursing assessment

       i) Perform thorough respiratory assessment.

      ii) Continuously measure oxygen saturation levels.

     iii) Monitor nutrition intake and fluid balance.

     iv) Observe for signs of infection.

    (b) Nursing diagnoses (same as section II,D,3,a,5,b of this chapter)

  (c) Nursing intervention
    i) Monitor respiratory status.
    ii) Administer oxygen as ordered.
    iii) Provide ventilator care.
    iv) Wean newborn from ventilator as tolerated.
    v) Provide adequate nutrition.
  (d) Nursing evaluation
    i) Newborn demonstrates adequate oxygenation.
    ii) Ventilator assistance is minimal.
    iii) Newborn remains free of infection.
    iv) Newborn maintains adequate hydration and gains weight.
    v) Parents understand infant's needs and increasingly participate in care.

4. Cardiac complications: patent ductus arteriosus
  a) Cause: Prematurity and low birth weight result in delay of normal spontaneous closure of the connection between the fetal aorta and pulmonary artery.
  b) Results: heart murmur, visible heart pulsation, tachycardia, tachypnea, possible hepatomegaly, and pulmonary edema
  c) Diagnosis: patency determined by aortic contrast echocardiography
  d) Essential nursing care for patent ductus arteriosus (same as section III,A,1,e of this chapter)

5. Neurologic complications: intraventricular hemorrhage (IVH)
  a) Causes: Birth asphyxia, hypotension, birth trauma resulting in hypoxia that enables rupture of cerebral blood vessels, mechanical ventilation
  b) Result: leading cause of neonatal death; impairment ranging from none to severe (grades III and IV associated with high degree of impairment)
  c) Diagnosis: Clinical signs range from none to marked change in condition: apnea, bradycardia, hypotension, seizures, decerebrate posturing; spinal fluid shows red cells; computed tomography and ultrasound can pinpoint location and size of hemorrhage.
  d) Medical management: Smaller hemorrhages resolve spontaneously; larger hemorrhages may require removal.
  e) Essential nursing care
    (1) Continuing observation of the newborn at risk
    (2) Monitoring for change in physical signs
    (3) Frequent measurement of head circumference and observation of fontanels for bulging
    (4) Providing supportive care to family as prognosis for severe IVH is very poor

6. Thermoregulatory complications: inability to maintain normal body temperature
   a) Causes: insufficient glycogen in the liver, insufficient brown fat stores, thin skin, high surface-to-mass ratio, inability to shiver, extended position of extremities
   b) Results: cold stress, metabolic acidosis, hypoglycemia
   c) Diagnosis: increased respirations and decrease in skin temperature
   d) Essential nursing care
      (1) Nursing assessment: Assess temperature with skin probe, and observe for signs of temperature loss.
      (2) Nursing diagnoses: high risk for injury (cold stress) related to immaturity of temperature-regulating mechanism; ineffective thermoregulation related to preterm status
      (3) Nursing intervention
         (a) Monitor temperature frequently.
         (b) Place infant in isolette or use radiant warmer, and periodically check heating unit temperature.
         (c) Maintain neutral thermal environment to minimize infant's oxygen consumption and to slow metabolism.
         (d) Warm transfusion blood, and warm and humidify oxygen.
      (4) Nursing evaluation
         (a) Infant maintains stable temperature.
         (b) Infant does not experience cold stress.
7. Gastrointestinal complications: inability to maintain adequate nutrition
   a) Causes
      (1) Mechanical feeding problems related to absent or weak sucking and swallowing reflexes
      (2) Decreased motility and absorption, incomplete digestion
   b) Results: limited ability to convert some essential amino acids to nonessential amino acids, inability to tolerate formula protein, decreased ability to tolerate saturated fats, decreased ability to digest lactose, calcium and phosphorus deficiencies, necrotizing enterocolitis
   c) Diagnosis: abdominal distention, gastric retention, vomiting, diarrhea, residual formula, metabolic acidosis, gastrointestinal bleeding, lethargy, irritability, apnea, unstable temperature, respiratory distress
   d) Medical management: Maintain fluid and electrolyte status; provide adequate nutrition; incorporate formula or breast milk into sterile water feedings slowly; use special formulas made for preterm newborns; use alternative feeding methods (gavage feeding, transpyloric nasojejunal or nasoduodenal tube feeding, gastrostomy, total parenteral nutrition [TPN]).

   e) Essential nursing care
      (1) Nursing assessment
         (a) Auscultate abdomen for bowel sounds; assess abdomen for appearance, tenderness, and girth.
         (b) Determine newborn's ability to suck and swallow and to tolerate oral intake.
      (2) Nursing diagnosis: altered nutrition, less than body requirements, related to inability to ingest and/or digest caloric requirements
      (3) Nursing intervention
         (a) Provide adequate calories; use method that best meets individual needs (breast, nipple, gavage, nasojejunal, gastrostomy, TPN).
         (b) Monitor weight daily.
         (c) Measure abdominal girth as needed.
         (d) Measure residual formula before tube feedings and replace.
         (e) Observe stool patterns and report any abnormalities.
         (f) Encourage parents to participate in feeding procedure.
         (g) Provide pacifier to suck on during gavage feeding to facilitate feeding.

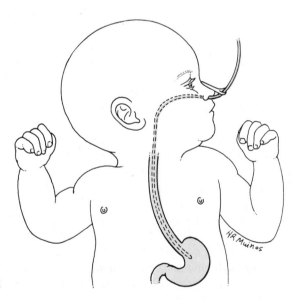

Figure 10-1
Gavage Feeding

(4) Nursing evaluation
    (a) Newborn adjusts to type of feeding.
    (b) Newborn maintains or gains weight.
    (c) Newborn maintains normal bowel movements.
8. Ocular complications: retinopathy of prematurity (ROP)
    a) Cause: unknown; occurs especially in low-birth-weight infants; believed to be related to oxygen administration in high concentrations, but other factors contribute to its development
    b) Result: dilation of retinal vessels and possible retinal detachment
    c) Diagnosis: fundal examination using indirect ophthalmoscope
    d) Medical management: transcleral cryotherapy (therapy that involves freezing scarred retinal vessels)
    e) Essential nursing care for retinopathy of prematurity: Provide parental support and education. Emphasis is on prevention—weaning infant from oxygen as quickly as tolerated.

III. Developmental disorders

A. Congenital defects
  1. Congenital heart defects
    a) Definition: heart disease that is present at birth
    b) Risk factors: environmental or genetic factors, maternal infection, maternal medication, substance or alcohol abuse, chromosomal abnormalities, positive family history
    c) Types
      (1) Acyanotic
        (a) Does not result in cyanosis
        (b) Examples: patent ductus arteriosus, atrial septal defect, ventricular septal defect
      (2) Cyanotic
        (a) Results in cyanosis
        (b) Examples: tetralogy of Fallot, transposition of great vessels, hypoplastic left heart syndrome
    d) Complications: possible congestive heart failure (CHF), pulmonary edema, failure to thrive
    e) Essential nursing care
      (1) Nursing assessment
        (a) Auscultate for heart murmur.
        (b) Observe for cyanosis and respiratory distress.
        (c) Observe peripheral pulses and capillary refill.
        (d) Monitor for signs of congestive heart failure: tachypnea, tachycardia, diaphoresis, hepatomegaly, and cardiomegaly.
        (e) Observe for feeding problems (e.g., frequent rest periods).
        (f) Listen for signs of stridor or choking.
        (g) Monitor weight gain.

See text pages
_____

        (2) Nursing diagnoses

            (a) Altered peripheral tissue perfusion related to decrease in circulating oxygen

            (b) Ineffective breathing pattern related to fatigue and congestive heart failure

            (c) Altered nutrition, less than body requirements, related to increased energy expenditure and difficulty coordinating breathing, sucking, and swallowing

            (d) Knowledge deficit (parental) related to lack of information about cardiac defect and implications

        (3) Nursing intervention

            (a) Provide humidified and warmed oxygen.

            (b) Monitor vital signs closely for signs of decompensation and congestive heart failure.

            (c) Monitor oxygen saturation levels.

            (d) Provide small, frequent feedings to avoid fatigue.

            (e) Chart fluid and nutritional intake and output.

            (f) Inform parents of newborn's condition, ongoing care, and treatment options.

            (g) Provide parents with information and support.

        (4) Nursing evaluation

            (a) Newborn's oxygen consumption and energy expenditure are minimal while at rest and feeding.

            (b) Parents are knowledgeable about the condition and their options and are able to verbalize their concerns.

    2. Cleft lip and cleft palate

      a) Definition: failure of soft or bony tissues of palate and upper jaw to close

      b) Risk factors: genetic factors, corticosteroid use, radiation, maternal infection, hypoxia in utero, dietary influences

      c) Types

        (1) Unilateral incomplete: cleft lip on one side

        (2) Unilateral complete: cleft lip and palate on one side

        (3) Bilateral complete: cleft lip and palate on both sides

      d) Complications: feeding problems resulting from inability to suck and swallow, aspiration of secretions, frequent respiratory tract infections, irregularities of the teeth, speech difficulties

      e) Essential nursing care

        (1) Nursing assessment: Assess newborn for extent of defect, ability to feed, and signs of respiratory distress.

        (2) Nursing diagnoses

            (a) Altered nutrition, less than body requirements, related to inability to suck and swallow effectively

(b) Ineffective airway clearance

(c) Knowledge deficit (parental) related to infant care

(d) High risk for dysfunctional grieving related to birth of infant with facial defect

(3) Nursing intervention

(a) Feed newborn in upright position to help swallowing and avoid aspiration.

(b) Use special nipple to accommodate oral cavity anomaly.

(c) Provide opportunity for family grieving and offer emotional support.

(d) Educate parents about condition, treatment options, special feeding considerations, and signs of airway obstruction.

(4) Nursing evaluation

(a) Newborn feeds adequately and gains weight.

(b) Parents understand the condition and verbalize their concerns, especially grief.

3. Hydrocephalus

a) Definition: excess accumulation of cerebrospinal fluid in ventricles of the brain resulting in head enlargement, "setting sun" appearance of the eyes, separated sutures, tense fontanels; often associated with spinal anomaly such as myelomeningocele

b) Risk factors: genetic and environmental influences

c) Complications: brain damage and infection

d) Essential nursing care

(1) Nursing assessment

(a) Measure head circumference daily.

(b) Assess daily for signs of increased intracranial pressure (e.g., widening fontanels and sutures, lethargy, irritability, vomiting).

(2) Nursing diagnoses

(a) Impaired skin integrity related to increased pressure

(b) High risk for infection related to limited motion and accumulation of fluid

(3) Nursing intervention

(a) Change position frequently, use sheepskin pillow, and keep skin clean and dry.

(b) Watch for signs of infection.

(c) Continue to monitor for signs of increased intracranial pressure.

(d) Prepare infant and parents for probable surgical intervention (shunt) to relieve pressure.

(4) Nursing evaluation

(a) Newborn's skin remains intact, and no infection develops.

(b) Changes in intracranial pressure are documented.

4. Tracheoesophageal fistula
   a) Definition: trachea abnormally joined to esophagus through fistula, causing excess mucus secretions, constant drooling, abdominal distention, and immediate regurgitation of feeding
   b) Risk factor: history of maternal polyhydramnios
   c) Complications: difficulty feeding and maintaining open airway; pneumonia; aspiration
   d) Essential nursing care
      (1) Nursing assessment
         (a) Check chart for history of polyhydramnios.
         (b) Observe for excessive mucus, drooling, and abdominal distention.
         (c) Assess tracheoesophageal patency at birth.
      (2) Nursing diagnoses
         (a) High risk for aspiration related to narrowed esophagus
         (b) High risk for infection related to aspirated gastric contents
      (3) Nursing intervention
         (a) Maintain open airway and prevent aspiration.
            i) Place on low intermittent suction.
            ii) Elevate head.
            iii) Suction accumulated secretions from mouth and nose every 15–30 minutes.
         (b) Monitor for signs of respiratory infection (e.g., tachypnea, chest retractions, cyanosis, rhonchi, rales).
         (c) Stabilize infant in preparation for surgical repair.
      (4) Nursing evaluation
         (a) Newborn does not aspirate secretions.
         (b) Newborn does not develop respiratory infection.

B. Genetic defects
   1. Down syndrome
      a) Definition: chromosomal abnormality (trisomy 21: most common type) resulting in low-set ears, single transverse palmar crease, large epicanthal folds
      b) Risk factor: maternal age
      c) Complications: cardiac defects, mental retardation, infection
      d) Essential nursing care for Down syndrome: Maintain fluid and electrolyte balance, prevent infection, provide oxygen therapy, provide support to parents, and encourage expression of feelings.
   2. Inborn errors of metabolism
      a) Definition: hereditary disorders transmitted by mutant genes; enzyme defect blocks metabolic path and results in accumulation of toxic metabolites

b) Risk factors: family history, northern European descent, decreased pigmentation

c) Types: phenylketonuria, maple syrup urine disease, galactosemia, homocystinuria

d) Complications: feeding problems, mental retardation, seizures, spasticity, opisthotonos, skeletal and ocular abnormalities, hepatosplenomegaly, jaundice

e) Essential nursing care

    (1) Nursing assessment

        (a) Identify at-risk newborns.

        (b) Observe newborn for signs of inborn error of metabolism.

    (2) Nursing diagnoses

        (a) Knowledge deficit (parental) related to special dietary management of inborn error in metabolism

        (b) Ineffective family coping related to parental guilt, secondary to hereditary nature of condition

    (3) Nursing intervention

        (a) Perform screening tests on newborn so that early intervention can be initiated.

        (b) Provide prompt dietary management.

        (c) Refer parents to centers that will provide information on dietary management.

    (4) Nursing evaluation

        (a) At-risk newborns are promptly identified.

        (b) Dietary management is initiated as soon as possible.

        (c) Parents are informed of community resources and use them.

1. Mrs. Alvarez is very upset because she cannot take her newborn son home. The newborn has been diagnosed with beta-hemolytic streptococcus infection and will need further hospitalization. Mrs. Alvarez asks the nurse, "How can this possibly happen here in a hospital?" The nurse explains that the newborn most likely acquired the infection from:

   a. A nurse with a cold.
   b. Contaminated food.
   c. A nonsterile needle injection.
   d. The birthing process itself.

2. Mrs. Alvarez asks the nurse if she and her husband can hold their baby. The nurse's best response is:

   a. "No, he needs to be in strict isolation."
   b. "You really shouldn't since you don't want to give him any more germs."
   c. "Only once a day, so healing can occur."
   d. "Yes, let me show you how."

3. Baby Girl S is born to an HIV-positive mother. An ELISA test done on the infant at 2 weeks of age shows positive HIV antibodies. This means that the infant:

   a. Has AIDS.
   b. Is HIV-positive.
   c. Has maternal HIV antibodies present.
   d. Will need further hospitalization and testing.

4. The nurse notes that Baby Girl S has small white patches on her tongue which, when scraped, cause bleeding. She identifies this as:

   a. *Chlamydia trachomatis.*
   b. *Staphylococcus aureus.*
   c. Herpes simplex virus.
   d. *Candida albicans.*

5. Baby Girl C is born to a heroin-addicted mother. Within 12 hours of birth, the baby begins to show signs of withdrawal. She shows extreme restless wakefulness, sneezing, and yawning. An appropriate nursing diagnosis related to these specific behavioral data is:

   a. Altered growth and development related to the effects of maternal substance abuse.
   b. Altered parenting related to newborn's hyperactivity.
   c. High risk for injury related to seizure activity.
   d. Altered sleep pattern disturbance related to central nervous system excitation.

6. A common effect of phototherapy that needs to be monitored by the nurse is:

   a. A positive Coombs' test.
   b. Diarrhea.
   c. Oliguria.
   d. Kernicterus.

7. The nurse is assessing a newborn born at 39 weeks. She observes loose, dry skin; sparse scalp hair; sunken abdomen; and insufficient subcutaneous fat. She identifies the newborn as:

   a. Small for gestational age (SGA).
   b. Large for gestational age (LGA).
   c. Appropriate for gestational age (AGA).
   d. Postterm.

8. Baby Boy M is born at 33 weeks' gestation. As a preterm infant, the most life-threatening risk for him is:

   a. Hyperthermia.
   b. Respiratory distress syndrome.
   c. Retinopathy of prematurity.
   d. Patent ductus arteriosus.

9. Baby Boy M needs to be gavage-fed. To accurately verify placement of gavage tube in the stomach prior to feeding, the nurse should:

a. Inject 5–10 cc of air and listen with stethoscope over epigastrium for sudden rush of air movement into stomach.

b. Place the end of the gavage tube in a glass of water and watch for air bubbles.

c. Obtain x-ray verification.

d. Aspirate for stomach contents with a syringe.

10. Baby Boy M is being monitored for apnea. When the pulse oximeter alarm goes off, the nurse should immediately:

a. Shake the isolette to stimulate the infant.

b. Observe the infant to see if he will breathe spontaneously.

c. Begin to administer oxygen.

d. Suction the nasopharynx.

11. Baby Boy A was born with a cleft lip and cleft palate. While doing parent teaching on proper feeding methods, the nurse instructs the parents to:

a. Feed the newborn in upright position with head and chest tilted slightly backward.

b. Place the newborn supine after feeding.

c. Use regular baby bottle nipple.

d. Anticipate an avid and eager feeder with few difficulties.

12. A client just delivered a baby boy with Apgar scores of 4 and 5 at 1 and 5 minutes. The mother asks the nurse, "What's going on? Why can't I see my baby?" The best response by the nurse is:

a. "It's nothing, really. I'll bring you the baby soon."

b. "Your son is having some difficulties breathing, and the pediatrician is with him."

c. "Just be patient. We'll give him to you as soon as possible."

d. "You have a nice baby boy."

1. **Correct answer is d.** Passage through the birth canal and vagina is the most likely way that the newborn acquired the infection.

a. It is possible that the infant acquired the infection from a nurse, but it is not as probable as during the birthing process.

b. Beta-hemolytic streptococci are not likely to be found in food.

c. It is unlikely that the infant acquired the infection from a nonsterile injection since needles are used only once.

2. **Correct answer is d.** Parental involvement is necessary. It does not affect the infection and may be helpful for the comfort and psychologic development of the infant. The nurse's response is correct and provides guidance to the parents.

a. The infant does not need to be in strict isolation.

b. This statement implies that the mother gave him the infection and might make her feel guilty.

c. Limiting the contact to once a day does not relate to healing or to the infection.

3. **Correct answer is c.** A 2-week-old infant's ELISA test indicates transmission of maternal antibodies. Testing should be repeated at 6 months of age.

a. An ELISA is not a definitive diagnostic test. There is a high percentage of false positives in the newborn. Also, the ELISA test indicates only that HIV antibodies are present but does not mean that AIDS is present.

b. There is no way to know at this age if the infant has been exposed to HIV. Studies indicate that 30%–50% of infants of HIV mothers are HIV-positive.

d. At this time, the infant would not need to be hospitalized.

4. Correct answer is d. *Candida albicans* causes thrush, an infection of the mouth that appears as small white patches. This is due to the fungus growth.

a. *Chlamydia* does not cause alterations in tongue mucosa. It most often affects a newborn's eyes.
b. Staphylococcus does not affect the oral mucosa as presented. It is commonly seen on the skin.
c. Herpes simplex virus does invade the oral mucosa. However, its lesions are not white patches.

5. Correct answer is d. Baby Girl C shows signs of altered sleep. This is caused by the effects of drug withdrawal on the central nervous system. A disturbed sleep-wake cycle is common in these children.

a, b, and **c.** Although any one of these diagnoses may apply to the heroin-addicted infant, the data presented about the infant's behavior support only answer d.

6. Correct answer is b. Diarrhea and watery stools are a common side effect of phototherapy. This is the result of increased bilirubin excretion.

a. A Coombs' test is done to determine whether the cause of jaundice is due to a hemolytic disease. It is not related to phototherapy.
c. Oliguria is not an effect of phototherapy.
d. Kernicterus is a complication of jaundice, resulting from bilirubin levels in brain cells; it is not an effect of phototherapy.

7. Correct answer is a. This baby shows signs of intrauterine growth retardation, a condition found in SGA babies.

b. An LGA newborn (one whose weight is above the 90th percentile on the intrauterine growth chart) would not have these characteristics.
c. An infant who is AGA would have characteristics of a normal newborn.
d. Postterm infants are those born after 42 weeks' gestation.

8. Correct answer is b. Respiratory distress syndrome (RDS) is a life-threatening disease for preterm infants. The lungs are not mature until 35 weeks' gestation, and mature alveoli are not present until 34–36 weeks. RDS is a leading cause of neonatal mortality.

a. Hyperthermia is not usually a threat in the preterm. More commonly, hypothermia is a life-threatening condition.
c. Retinopathy of prematurity is an acquired disease in the preterm infant. It is not life-threatening.
d. A patent ductus arteriosus will present symptoms by the third day of life. Closure can be completed by medical therapy, medications, or surgical corrections. There may be long-term complications.

9. Correct answer is d. Aspiration of stomach contents is an acceptable method of verifying gavage tube placement. If there is any question about gastric contents, the aspirate can be tested for pH.

a. This is far too much air to inject into a preterm infant's stomach; 2–4 cc should be sufficient.
b. This method is incorrect since the stomach often has air in it as well as the lungs.
c. An x-ray verification is unwarranted; there is a medical risk of x-ray exposure.

10. Correct answer is b. When the apnea alarm sounds, the nurse should first observe the infant to evaluate spontaneous return to breathing. Preterm infants have many apneic periods, which are thought to relate to neural immaturity.

a. Stimulation by rubbing the infant's feet, ankles, or back would be the next step if Baby Boy M did not breathe spontaneously.
c and **d.** Suctioning and administration of oxygen would be the next steps to control dyspnea and cyanosis. If the infant still did not respond, it would be appropriate to begin ventilation by bag and mask.

11. **Correct answer is a.** This method of feeding aids in swallowing and prevents aspiration.

   b. The supine position would be inappropriate since the newborn could aspirate feedings and secretions.
   c. Newborns with cleft lip and palate need to have special nipples that fill the cleft and allow sucking.
   d. Parents need to be prepared for long, frustrating feeding times.

12. **Correct answer is b.** Parents have a need to know what is happening. A truthful and honest response is best.

   a. This answer is dishonest and minimizes the parents' concern.
   c. This answer does not provide support to the parents and is scolding in nature.
   d. Although a true statement, it does not respond to the mother's question.

11

Normal Postpartum Period

NURSING HIGHLIGHTS

1. Nursing in the postpartal period includes both physical and psychologic caregiving and client teaching.
2. Maternal physiologic changes begin immediately after delivery; restoration of the prepregnancy state usually occurs within 2–3 months.
3. Nurse teaches client both evaluation and self-care skills so that she can continue these measures after discharge.
4. Anticipatory guidance from the nurse during the role transition to parenthood can head off potential problems.
5. The maternity nurse's skill and knowledge helps the family in bonding and developing attachment.

GLOSSARY

attachment—gradual development of maternal-infant emotional bonding
en face position—position in which client holds infant face to face, and eye contact is sustained
engrossment—gradual development of paternal-infant emotional bonding

introitus—entrance into canal or cavity
thrombophlebitis—inflammation of the wall of a vein and the formation of a
   blood clot

ENHANCED OUTLINE

I. Maternal physiologic changes and adaptations

See text pages

A. Reproductive organs
   1. Uterus
      a) Uterine involution: rapid reduction in size and return to
         prepregnancy state (puerperium: period between birth of child
         and complete involution of uterus)
         (1) After placental expulsion, uterus contracts to size of
             grapefruit.
             (a) Firm consistency is normal.
             (b) Boggy, or soft, consistency (uterine atony) is associated
                 with hemorrhage (same as section I,A of Chapter 12).
         (2) Fundus descends into pelvis at a rate of 1–2 cm a day.
         (3) Uterus reaches nonpregnant size by 4–6 weeks.
         (4) Falling estrogen and progesterone levels contribute to
             involution.
         (5) Afterpains are periodic uterine contractions of varying
             intensity.
             (a) More common in multiparas
             (b) Stimulated by oxytocin
                 i) Endogenous oxytocin: released by pituitary gland;
                    release enhanced in response to nipple stimulation
                    from breastfeeding
                 ii) Exogenous oxytocin: administered by injection to aid
                     involution
      b) Lochia: postdelivery uterine discharge consisting of blood, tissue,
         and mucus
         (1) Increases with ambulation and breastfeeding
         (2) Characterized as rubra, serosa, or alba, depending on
             components (see Nurse Alert, "Characteristics of Lochia")
         (3) Ceases by third week postpartum
   2. Cervix
      a) Cervix shortens and becomes thicker and firmer by 24 hours.
      b) Cervix heals completely by 6–12 weeks.
      c) Round os of nullipara may appear as a transverse slit after
         childbirth.
   3. Vagina
      a) Introitus is erythematous and edematous; it subsides by 2 weeks.
      b) Vaginal lubrication is decreased and mucosa is thinner; it returns
         to normal when menstruation resumes.

    c) Vagina is edematous; it returns to smaller (although not prepregnant) size by 6–8 weeks.

  4. Pelvic musculature

    a) Injury during childbirth causes a weakening of muscular and fascial supports.

    b) Pelvic muscle exercises (Kegel exercises) can help pelvic musculature regain strength.

  5. Abdomen

    a) Abdominal wall returns to prepregnant state by 6 weeks.

    b) Diastasis recti abdominis is a separation of the muscles of the abdominal wall from overdistention; it is not uncommon, especially after multiple births and cesarean sections.

! NURSE *ALERT* !

Characteristics of Lochia

Normal characteristics
- Lochia rubra: 1–3 days postpartum
  - —Bright red
  - —Bloody
  - —May have small clots
  - —Heavy to moderate flow
  - —Musty, inoffensive odor
- Lochia serosa: 4–7 days postpartum
  - —Pink to brown
  - —No clots
  - —Decrease in flow
  - —No odor
- Lochia alba: 1–3 weeks postpartum
  - —Cream-colored or yellowish
  - —Scant flow
  - —No odor

Warning signs
- Blood spurts from vagina.
- Heavy bleeding persists or returns after lochia rubra; this may be sign of hemorrhage.
- Foul-smelling discharge occurs; this may be sign of infection.
- Large clots are present.

B. Breasts
  1. Colostrum (substance high in protein and antibodies that precedes breast milk) is secreted for several days.
  2. Nipple tenderness may be evident for 48–72 hours after delivery; it is accompanied by breast tenderness in first few days to a week after breastfeeding begins. "Toughening" of nipples develops in time.
  3. Engorgement (swelling and vasocongestion of breasts) can occur.
  4. In breastfeeding clients, breast milk follows colostrum by day 3 or 4.
  5. In clients who are not breastfeeding, lactation ceases within a week.

C. Endocrine system
  1. Placental hormones
     a) Human placental lactogen (hPL) and human chorionic gonadotropin (hCG) levels decline rapidly.
     b) Estrogen and progesterone levels decline.
     c) Progesterone production begins with first postpartum ovulation.
  2. Pituitary hormones
     a) Serum levels of prolactin are influenced by number of times per day breastfeeding occurs.
     b) Levels of follicle stimulating hormone (FSH) drop immediately after childbirth and rise slowly to normal levels by week 3.
     c) Luteinizing hormone (LH) levels rise after first postpartum ovulation occurs.
  3. Resumption of ovulation and menstruation
     a) Nonbreastfeeding clients: 70% resume menstruation by 12 weeks. Ovulation may precede menstruation.
     b) Breastfeeding clients: 45% resume menstruation by 12 weeks.
        (1) Variability of return of menstruation and ovulation results from differences in breastfeeding and from individual hormonal levels.
        (2) Breastfeeding is not an effective birth control method.

D. Cardiovascular system
  1. Blood volume
     a) Increases approximately 40% during pregnancy
     b) Returns to prepregnancy levels by week 3 or 4
  2. Vital signs and blood pressure
     a) Orthostatic hypotension may occur for 48 hours.
     b) Bradycardia (40–50 beats per minute) may occur for 6–10 days.
     c) Elevated blood pressure may be an indication of pregnancy-induced hypertension (PIH) and should be monitored closely.
  3. Blood constituents
     a) Transient increase in hematocrit related to hemoconcentration; returns to prepregnancy level by week 4 or 5
     b) Increase in leukocyte level: 20,000–25,000/mm^3; returns to prepregnancy level by day 10–12
     c) Extensive activation of blood-clotting factors; increases risk of thromboembolisms, varicosities, and hemorrhoids; returns to prepregnancy levels within a few days

E. Gastrointestinal system
   1. Appetite increases shortly after delivery.
   2. Constipation is common.
   3. Weight loss occurs.
      a) Loss of up to 10–12 lb immediately after birth (fetus, placenta, amniotic fluid, blood loss)
      b) Loss of 5 lb during early puerperium
      c) Return to prepregnancy weight by 6–8 weeks postpartum (if client gained the average of 25–30 lb)

F. Urinary system
   1. Diuresis: Urinary output increases during early postpartal period.
   2. Diaphoresis: Sweating increases during puerperium, especially at night.
   3. Birth-induced trauma to urethra and bladder
      a) Results in overdistention, incomplete bladder emptying, and buildup of residual urine
      b) Increases risk of urinary tract infection (same as section I,C of Chapter 12)
      c) Increases risk of hematuria (which may be confused with lochial components)

G. Neurologic system: Puerperal changes involve reversals of pregnancy- and labor-induced conditions.
   1. Pregnancy-induced conditions: carpal tunnel syndrome, numbness and tingling of fingers and thighs, and leg cramps, which resolve following delivery; headache and hypertonic deep tendon reflexes (from PIH), which vary in duration
   2. Labor-induced condition: headache (from leakage of cerebrospinal fluid during placement of needle for spinal anesthesia), which varies in duration

H. Musculoskeletal system
   1. Joints stabilize within 6–8 weeks.
   2. Center of gravity and posture return to prepregnancy state following delivery.

See text pages

II. Maternal (and familial) psychologic changes and adaptations

A. Development of attachment
   1. Linear process that ensures child's mental and physical well-being
   2. Maternal behaviors enhancing attachment
      a) Feelings of warmth, affection, and protectiveness
      b) Caregiving knowledge and skills (diapering, feeding, and bathing, using en face position)

3. Paternal behaviors enhancing attachment: sense of absorption, preoccupation, and engrossment
4. Attachment of siblings and others
    a) Newborns are capable of bonding with more than 1 individual.
    b) Sibling acceptance must be promoted and sibling rivalry managed by parents.
5. Factors that influence attachment
    a) Physical condition of parent or infant
    b) Parents' emotional health
    c) Family's social support system
    d) Communication and caregiving skills
    e) Parental proximity to the infant
    f) Parent-infant fit

B. Attainment of maternal role: progressive process
    1. Anticipatory stage: During pregnancy, client observes role models, especially own mother.
    2. Formal stage: At birth of child, client acts as she believes others expect her to, follows suggestions, and is hesitant; this is also called "taking-in" period.
    3. Informal stage: Client begins making her own mothering decisions; this is also called "taking-hold" period.
    4. Personal stage: Client has become comfortable with the idea of herself as a mother and her unique interaction with her child.

III. Essential nursing care

A. Nursing assessment
    1. Risk factors
        a) Identify maternal risk factors.
            (1) Pregnancy-induced hypertension
            (2) Diabetes
            (3) Heart disease
            (4) Substance abuse
        b) Identify gestation-related risk factors.
            (1) Overdistention of uterus (multiple gestation or hydramnios)
            (2) Abruptio placentae
            (3) Placenta previa
            (4) Preterm labor
        c) Identify labor-related risk factors.
            (1) Difficult birth
            (2) Precipitous or prolonged labor
            (3) Cesarean delivery
            (4) Prolonged period of time in stirrups
        d) Identify postpartum risk factors: retained placenta or uterine atony.

See text pages
_____

2. Vital signs
   a) Assess vital signs at regular intervals.
   b) Alteration in vital signs may be a sign of complication. A temperature >100.6°F after first 24 hours warrants investigation (a possible sign of infection).
3. Reproductive/genitourinary systems
   a) Check progress of involution (see Nurse Alert, "Factors that Retard Uterine Involution").
      (1) Determine fundal height and position and uterine consistency.
         (a) Measure fundal height by fingerbreadths in relation to umbilicus.
         (b) Check that fundus is positioned in midline.
         (c) Check that uterus is of firm consistency, not boggy.
      (2) Assess character and amount of lochia: color, odor, and presence of blood clots.
   b) Determine if bladder is distended.
4. Lower extremities: assess for thrombophlebitis (see also Chapter 12, section I,E).
5. Gastrointestinal system
   a) Inquire about bowel movement and passage of gas.

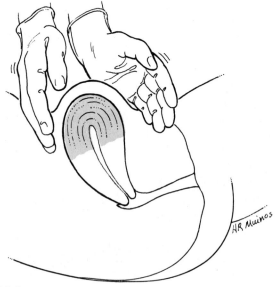

Figure 11-1
Fundal Massage

    b) Auscultate for bowel sounds.

    c) Palpate for abdominal distention.

6. Perineum

    a) Observe and palpate for signs of complications: hematoma, bruising, edema, redness, or tenderness.

    b) Inspect episiotomy site for signs of infection.

    c) Inspect for hemorrhoids.

7. Breasts

    a) Assess breast size, shape, color, symmetry, consistency, and tenderness; check nipples for cracks.

    b) Assess changes in size, consistency, and temperature once breastfeeding has been initiated.

8. Laboratory evaluations

    a) Obtain hematocrit and hemoglobin to test for anemia.

    b) Obtain samples for white blood count.

    c) Obtain urine for urinalysis.

    d) Obtain direct Coombs' test if mother is Rh negative to determine need for prophylactic Rh_o (D) immune globulin (RhoGAM).

9. Psychosocial factors

    a) Assess reaction to the childbirth process.

    b) Assess attitude toward infant and indications of attachment.

    c) Assess adaptations to caregiving responsibilities and transition to maternal role.

    d) Assess family interactions.

    e) Assess knowledge of self-care and infant-care practices.

    f) Assess availability of support systems (father and other relatives).

    g) Acknowledge cultural variations.

B. Nursing diagnoses

  1. Constipation related to decreased bowel motility and abdominal muscle tone, dehydration, and painful defecation

  2. Altered urinary elimination related to postpartum diuresis and urinary retention

I. Maternal physiologic changes and adaptations	II. Maternal (and familial) psychologic changes and adaptations	III. Essential nursing care

3. Pain related to afterpains, episiotomy, hemorrhoids, breast engorgement, and breastfeeding
4. Impaired skin integrity related to laceration, episiotomy, and cesarean birth
5. High risk for infection related to impaired skin integrity and tissue trauma
6. Fluid volume deficit related to decreased intake and blood loss
7. Sleep pattern disturbances related to discomfort and infant feeding
8. Knowledge deficit related to self-care, infant care, and health maintenance
9. Situational low self-esteem related to knowledge deficits, "baby blues," and change in role identities
10. Family coping: potential for growth as infant is integrated into family

C. Nursing intervention
1. Uterine atony (see Nurse Alert, "Procedure for Assessing and Massaging the Uterus")
2. Full urinary bladder
   a) Help client to empty bladder spontaneously as soon as possible after birth (assist to bathroom or onto a bedpan and use techniques to initiate voiding: running water, sitz bath, pouring water on perineum).
   b) Palpate bladder after delivery to determine whether complete emptying occurred.
   c) Encourage fluid intake.
   d) Determine whether sterile catheterization is required.
3. Episiotomy or lacerations
   a) Position client on side and inspect perineum.
   b) Apply ice pack for first 24 hours.

! NURSE *ALERT* !

Procedure for Assessing and Massaging the Uterus

- Have client void prior to assessment.
- Position client on back.
- Use one hand to support lower fundus above pubic bone and the other hand to measure distance in fingerbreadths between top of fundus and umbilicus.
- Determine uterine consistency.
- Stimulate uterine tone by gently massaging the fundus until firm; express clots.
- If uterus remains boggy, notify physician or nurse-midwife. Anticipate administration of oxytocin or prostaglandin to control bleeding and stimulate uterine contractions.

Measures for Perineal Self-Care

Encourage client to:

✔ Lie on side or sit on pillow.
✔ Apply ice pack, topical anesthetic, witch hazel, or moist or dry heat for pain.
✔ Use squeeze bottle with warm water after using toilet.
✔ Clean area regularly in shower or sitz bath.
✔ Pat dry from front to back using tissue.

    c) Apply moist heat (sitz bath) and/or dry heat (heat lamp) after first 24 hours.

    d) Educate client on perineal care techniques (see Client Teaching Checklist, "Measures for Perineal Self-Care").

  4. Breasts

    a) Lactation suppression

      (1) Educate client on lactation suppression techniques (see Client Teaching Checklist, "Lactation Suppression Techniques").

      (2) Administer medication as ordered (bromocriptine [Parlodel]).

        (a) Medication prevents secretion of prolactin (hormone that stimulates lactation).

        (b) Rebound breast engorgement may occur when medication is discontinued.

        (c) Bromocriptine is contraindicated in client who is hypertensive.

    b) Breast care during lactation

      (1) Educate client on care of the breasts during lactation (see Client Teaching Checklist, "Care of the Breasts during Lactation").

Lactation Suppression Techniques

Recommendations for client:

✔ Wear properly fitting support bra or breast binder.
✔ Avoid breast stimulation: infant sucking, hand or pump expressing, and water stream from shower.
✔ Place ice packs on breasts to alleviate engorgement.
✔ Take medication (bromocriptine) as prescribed for either 14 or 21 days.

I. Maternal physiologic changes and adaptations	II. Maternal (and familial) psychologic changes and adaptations	III. Essential nursing care

(2) Advise client to wear a well-fitting bra that provides support and maintains breast shape.
   (a) Straps should be cloth and easily adjustable.
   (b) Back should be wide with at least 3 rows of hooks for adjustment.

5. Afterpains
   a) Educate client on cause and purpose of afterpains, and provide reassurance that they are normal.
   b) Teach self-care measures, such as emptying the bladder, using a heating pad, lying on stomach, and performing leg-lift exercises.
   c) Offer pain medication as ordered to promote comfort.

6. Thrombophlebitis
   a) Inform client to avoid constricting garters or clothing.
   b) Provide information on warning signs of thrombophlebitis (see Client Teaching Checklist, "Signs of Thrombosis and Infection").
   c) Encourage early and frequent ambulation.

7. Sexuality and contraception: Inform client that:
   a) Intercourse may be resumed after episiotomy has healed and lochial flow has stopped.
   b) Vaginal dryness may require lubrication.
   c) Milk may be secreted during orgasm.
   d) Fatigue, low hormone levels, and adjusting to maternal role may adversely affect sexual desire.
   e) Return of ovulation is variable; contraception is necessary if couple wish to avoid pregnancy.

✔ CLIENT TEACHING CHECKLIST ✔

Care of the Breasts during Lactation

Recommendations for client:

✔ Wash breasts with plain water during daily bath or shower.
✔ Avoid using soap on the nipples.
✔ Keep nipples dry.
✔ Expose nipples to air for 15–30 minutes each day.
✔ Allow breast milk to dry on the nipples for natural soothing and antiseptic properties.
✔ Inspect nipples daily to detect any cracks or blisters.
✔ Avoid using ointments and creams on the nipples.

8. Postpartum "baby blues" (same as section II,A of Chapter 12)
   a) Provide opportunity for client to express her feelings.
   b) Offer empathetic listening and support.
9. Psychologic adaptation and parental attachment
   a) Reinforce positive behaviors.
   b) Provide appropriate teaching and guidance.
10. Health maintenance
    a) Stress importance of obtaining adequate nutrition.
       (1) Encourage client to increase fluid intake (a glass of fluid every hour while awake).
       (2) Recommend that breastfeeding client maintain intake of nutrients at pregnancy levels and increase caloric intake by 200 calories over pregnancy levels.
       (3) Encourage breastfeeding client to avoid caffeine and gas-forming foods.
    b) Stress importance of getting adequate rest and sleep.
       (1) Inform client that rest periods or naps are essential.
       (2) Inform client that sleep deprivation may exacerbate other stresses.
    c) Help client identify support system for helping with household chores.
    d) Provide information on bathing.
       (1) Inform client that showering is permitted within a few hours of delivery (may be delayed for a day if regional anesthesia was used).
       (2) Inform client that tub baths should be postponed until lochia stops.
    e) Provide information on relief of constipation.
       (1) Advise client to increase intake of fluids and roughage.
       (2) Recommend that client take stool softener or laxative (breastfeeding client should check laxative choice with physician because some are excreted in breast milk).
    f) Provide information on resumption of exercises and activity level.
       (1) Encourage client to gradually begin simple exercises in the hospital and continue at home.

(2) Advise client to avoid heavy lifting and strenuous exercises for 4–5 weeks.

(3) Advise client to stop performing exercise or activity if lochial flow increases or pain results.

    11. Preparation for discharge

        a) Provide written information, referrals, and telephone numbers for community resources.

        b) Arrange for follow-up appointment.

        c) Educate client on possible danger signs (see Client Teaching Checklist, "Postpartum Danger Signs").

D. Nursing evaluation

    1. Uterus is contracting and lochial flow is moderate.

    2. Client voids adequate amounts of urine and has a bowel elimination without difficulty.

    3. Episiotomy is healing without signs of infection, and perineal pain is absent or minimal.

    4. Lactation is successfully suppressed, or breastfeeding is successfully initiated.

    5. Client understands need for balanced diet and increased fluids, sleep, and rest periods.

    6. Client understands signs of infection and that they must be reported promptly.

    7. Signs of infection are absent.

✔ CLIENT TEACHING CHECKLIST ✔

Postpartum Danger Signs

Tell client to report these signs to a physician immediately:

✔ Heavy vaginal bleeding
✔ Increased or foul-smelling vaginal discharge
✔ Recurrence of bright-red bleeding
✔ Fever, with or without chills
✔ Swollen, tender, red, or hot area on leg
✔ Burning or pain with urination
✔ Inability to urinate
✔ Persistent pelvic or perineal pain
✔ Swollen, tender, red, or hot area on breast
✔ Persistent feelings of depression or lack of interest in self or baby

8. Client understands postpartum "baby blues."
9. Client gradually increases exercise and activity levels and plans to continue exercising after discharge.
10. Client and partner understand aspects of postpartal sexual activity and the need for contraception.
11. Client interacts positively with newborn and demonstrates acceptance of maternal role.
12. Parents describe plans for infant care at home and include other family members.
13. Parents verbalize their concerns but also feel competent in roles as parents.

1. Postpartum uterine involution can best be described as:

   a. Relaxation of uterine muscles with subsequent shedding of uterine wall.
   b. Uterine changes due to contraction of the uterus, autolysis of the uterine wall, and endometrial regeneration.
   c. Atrophy of uterine cells and hyperplasia of endometrium, facilitated by increased circulatory levels of estrogen and progesterone.
   d. Release of proteolytic enzymes that dissolve the excess uterine tissues with subsequent uterine hyperplasia.

2. Angela has delivered a healthy 7-lb baby boy vaginally with no complications. On day 3 postpartum, the nurse is giving Angela predischarge teaching. For which of the following conditions should the nurse instruct Angela to notify her caregiver immediately?

   a. Fatigue
   b. Constipation
   c. Bright-red vaginal bleeding
   d. Perineal pain

3. Which of the following postpartum women is most likely to experience afterpains?

   a. Patrice, age 23, gravida 3 para 3, breastfeeding
   b. Martha, age 30, gravida 1 para 1, breastfeeding, type I diabetes
   c. Marguerite, age 42, gravida 1 para 1, taking bromocriptine (Parlodel)
   d. Janice, age 16, gravida 2 para 2, bottlefeeding, cesarean delivery

4. Immediately after delivery, a woman can expect weight loss. The usual weight loss is:

   a. 5–6 lb.
   b. 7–8 lb.
   c. 10–12 lb.
   d. 15 lb or more.

5. Mrs. Kline delivered a healthy 7-lb baby boy vaginally with no complications and was transferred to the postpartum unit. Four hours after delivery, the nurse assesses Mrs. Kline's uterus to be 2 fingerbreadths above the umbilicus and to the right. The nurse should first:

   a. Initiate fundal massage.
   b. Assess for full bladder.
   c. Monitor vital signs every 15 minutes.
   d. Assess character and amount of lochia.

6. Mrs. Kline states to the nurse, "I feel so weak and tired. I must have lost a lot of blood during delivery." The nurse answers, "Your blood loss was normal, but the process of labor tires most women." The nurse's response is based on the knowledge that normal blood loss during a vaginal delivery is:

   a. Less than 100 ml.
   b. 400–500 ml.
   c. 1000 ml.
   d. 1500 ml or more.

7. Mrs. Kline has decided not to breastfeed her infant. An appropriate nursing action to facilitate suppression of lactation is:

   a. Manual expression of milk.
   b. Application of moist heat.
   c. Restriction of oral fluids.
   d. Use of ice packs.

8. Mrs. Kline is to be given bromocriptine (Parlodel) to suppress lactation. A maternal side effect of which the nurse must be aware is:

   a. Hypotension.
   b. Thromboembolic disease.
   c. Constipation.
   d. Hirsutism.

9. When Mrs. Kline is 2 days postpartum, the nurse would expect fundal height to be:

   a. At the umbilicus.
   b. 1 fingerbreadth below umbilicus.
   c. 2 fingerbreadths below umbilicus.
   d. 3 fingerbreadths below umbilicus.

10. Prior to discharge, the nurse notes that Mrs. Kline's rubella titer is 1:8. Mrs. Kline will be advised to:

   a. Have a rubella vaccination before discharge.

   b. Obtain a rubella vaccination at her 6-week checkup.

   c. Have no vaccine because she is immune to rubella.

   d. Have the titer level repeated.

11. The nurse observes Mr. Kline holding and talking to his son and being generally preoccupied with his child. This is called:

   a. Engrossment.

   b. Mutuality.

   c. Entrainment.

   d. Biorhythmicity.

12. A postpartum client asks the nurse when she and her partner can resume sexual intercourse. The nurse's response should be:

   a. "Sexual activity can resume after your 6-week checkup."

   b. "As soon as your episiotomy site is healed, you can resume intercourse."

   c. "Sexual activity can begin when vaginal discharge has stopped and the episiotomy is healed."

   d. "Sexual activity can begin as soon as you feel up to it."

ANSWERS

1. **Correct answer is b.** Involution begins after delivery with a rapid decrease in the size of the uterus. This is done by uterine contractions and an autolytic process whereby protein material of the uterine wall is broken down and absorbed. At the same time, endometrial regeneration occurs in the decidua basalis.

   a. The uterine muscles do not relax after delivery.

   c. Uterine cells do atrophy after delivery. However, estrogen and progesterone rapidly decrease after delivery.

   d. Proteolytic enzymes are released, promoting autolysis, and subsequently the uterine wall is broken down and absorbed. However, there is no hyperplasia at this time.

2. **Correct answer is c.** Bright-red vaginal bleeding (lochia rubra) is present days 1–3 postpartum. A return to lochia rubra may indicate hemorrhage.

   a and b. Fatigue and constipation are common occurrences in postpartum women and do not require notification of caregiver.

   d. Perineal pain is common for women who have had a vaginal delivery. The caregiver does not need to be notified.

3. **Correct answer is a.** When the infant sucks during breastfeeding, oxytocin is released. Oxytocin causes contractions of the uterine muscles. Multiparity is also an indicator for afterpains.

   b. A gravida 1 para 1 does not usually experience afterpains because she has increased muscle tone. Also, diabetes is not a predictor for afterpains.

   c. A primipara usually does not experience afterpains since she has increased muscle tone. Also, bromocriptine suppresses lactation and corresponding oxytocin release. Age is not a factor.

   d. This client would not experience the uterine contractions caused by release of oxytocin as she is bottle-feeding. Also, a cesarean delivery is not an indicator for afterpains.

4. **Correct answer is c.** Immediately after delivery, a weight loss of 10–12 lb corresponds to fetus and placenta, amniotic fluid, and blood loss. An additional 5–8 lb during the first weeks postpartum is due to perspiration and diuresis.

   a, b, and **d.** All are incorrect based on the information given in correct answer c.

5. **Correct answer is b.** A full bladder can displace the uterus and interfere with effective uterine contractions.

   a. If a full bladder is not the problem, the nurse should then initiate fundal massage.
   c. By the fourth hour after delivery, vital signs can be taken every 4 hours.
   d. Although lochia assessment is routine every 4 hours, the bladder distention may well be the cause of Mrs. Kline's uterine height and softness.

6. **Correct answer is b.** Normal blood loss during a vaginal delivery is approximately 400–500 ml.

   a. A blood loss of less than 100 ml would be very unusual.
   c and d. A blood loss of 1000 ml or 1500 ml or more with a vaginal delivery would indicate a complication. With a cesarean section, blood loss may be 1000 ml or more.

7. **Correct answer is d.** Application of ice packs and subsequent vasoconstriction will facilitate suppression of lactation.

   a and b. These measures would facilitate breastfeeding and milk production.
   c. Restriction of oral fluids would be contraindicated in any postpartum woman due to increased diaphoresis during postpartum.

8. **Correct answer is a.** Hypotension is the primary side effect for which the nurse must watch. Thus the drug should be delayed until maternal vital signs are stable.

   b. There does not seem to be a problem with thromboembolic disease with the use of bromocriptine as would be seen when giving estrogen-based medications such as chlorotrianisene (TACE).
   c and d. Constipation and hirsutism are not side effects of bromocriptine.

9. **Correct answer is c.** Normal fundal height decreases 1 fingerbreadth (1 cm) each day postpartum. At day 2 postpartum, Mrs. Kline should have a fundal height 2 fingerbreadths below the umbilicus.

   a. At delivery, the fundus is at the umbilicus.
   b. At day 1 postpartum, fundal height is 1 fingerbreadth below umbilicus.
   d. At day 3 postpartum, fundal height is 3 fingerbreadths below umbilicus.

10. **Correct answer is a.** A rubella titer of 1:8 or less indicates that Mrs. Kline is serologically negative and needs to have rubella vaccination prior to discharge.

    b. She should not wait for her 6-week checkup to receive immunization because she could be pregnant by then, putting the fetus at risk for rubella.
    c. This answer is incorrect for reason given in correct answer a.
    d. There is no need to repeat the titer level at this time.

11. **Correct answer is a.** *Engrossment* is a term used to describe paternal behaviors that enhance attachment.

    b. *Mutuality* refers to infant behaviors and characteristics and corresponding maternal behaviors and characteristics.
    c. Movement by an infant in time with adult speech is called *entrainment*.
    d. *Biorhythmicity* refers to the infant's ability to establish a personal rhythm.

12. **Correct answer is c.** Intercourse can resume as soon as lochia has stopped and the episiotomy is healed.

    a. There is no need to wait for the 6-week checkup if lochia has stopped.
    b. While it is true that intercourse can be resumed once the episiotomy site is healed, the lochia should also be absent.
    d. This is an inappropriate response because intercourse should not be resumed until lochia has ceased.

12

Complications during Postpartum Period

NURSING HIGHLIGHTS

1. Nurse plays a major role in the identification and prevention of postpartal complications.
2. Early hospital discharge requires that the client be taught the signs and symptoms of hemorrhage, infection, mastitis, thromboembolism, failure to bond, and depression.
3. Because postpartal complications can have a negative effect on the maternal-infant attachment process, nurse must be especially vigilant in promoting bonding between client who has postpartal complication and her infant.
4. The nurse's role is critical in the case of perinatal death; an understanding of grieving will allow nurse to help families cope with the loss.

GLOSSARY

hemoptysis—expectoration of blood-tinged mucus
vesicoureteral reflux—a backward flow of urine from the bladder into a ureter

ENHANCED OUTLINE

See text pages

I. Physical problems

A. Hemorrhage
1. Definition: blood loss >500 ml caused by uterine atony (relaxation of the uterus), retained placental fragments, or blood coagulation problems
2. Types
   a) Early hemorrhage: occurs within the first 24 hours of delivery
   b) Late hemorrhage: occurs more than 24 hours after delivery
3. Risk factors: overdistention of the uterus; grand multiparity; use of operative obstetrics; use of oxytocin or anesthesia that relaxes the uterus; history of hemorrhage, uterine infection, or fibroids; placenta previa; abruptio placentae
4. Medical therapy: fundal massage, bimanual compression of the uterus (compression of the uterus by placing one hand on the abdomen and one hand inside the vagina), administration of medication to control bleeding and stimulate uterine contractions, curettage (scraping of the inside of the uterus), blood and/or fluid replacement, possible hysterectomy
5. Essential nursing care
   a) Nursing assessment
      (1) Assess prenatal history and perinatal events to identify at-risk clients.
      (2) Observe for signs of hemorrhage (see Nurse Alert, "Signs of Postpartal Hemorrhage").
      (3) Document amount of bleeding.
   b) Nursing diagnoses
      (1) Fluid volume deficit related to blood loss
      (2) Anxiety related to lack of control over unforeseen complication
   c) Nursing intervention
      (1) Check fundal height and consistency, and provide fundal massage as needed.
      (2) Check for evidence of excessive bleeding.
      (3) Monitor blood loss.
      (4) Provide fluid replacement and medications to correct uterine atony.
      (5) Observe for signs of anemia and monitor hematocrit.
      (6) Provide information about the condition: its causes, consequences, and treatment.

      (7) Encourage client to express concerns about effects of the complication on parenting.

  d) Nursing evaluation

      (1) Signs of hemorrhage are detected early and managed effectively.

      (2) Client understands the condition and expresses concerns.

B. Infection of the reproductive tract

  1. Definition: contamination of reproductive tract by bacteria

  2. Types

    a) Localized infections: infection related to episiotomy, laceration, wound

    b) Endometritis (metritis): infection of the endometrium at the placental site

    c) Pelvic cellulitis (parametritis): infection of the connective tissue in the pelvis

    d) Peritonitis: infection of the peritoneum

  3. Risk factors

    a) Labor-related factors: chorioamnionitis, cesarean birth after onset of labor, premature rupture of membranes, multiple internal examinations, prolonged labor, laceration, episiotomy

    b) Non–labor-related factors: anemia, poor nutritional status, lack of prenatal care, sexual intercourse after rupture of membranes, underlying disease, immunosuppression, obesity

  4. Medical therapy: antibiotics, sitz bath, analgesics, wound drainage

  5. Essential nursing care

    a) Nursing assessment

      (1) Assess prenatal history for factors predisposing to infection or retarded wound healing.

      (2) Inspect perineum for signs of infection: *r*edness, *e*dema, *e*cchymosis, *d*ischarge, *a*pproximation of wound edges (REEDA).

      (3) Check for fever (>100.6°F after first 24 hours), chills, pain, and foul-smelling lochia.

      b) Nursing diagnoses

        (1) High risk for injury related to spread of infection

        (2) Pain related to presence of infection

        (3) Altered parenting related to delayed parent-infant attachment

      c) Nursing intervention

        (1) Promote wound healing with sitz baths, appropriate perineal care, diet enriched with protein and vitamin C, increased fluid intake, and early ambulation.

        (2) Monitor vital signs and progress of therapy.

        (3) Administer antibiotics as ordered.

        (4) Provide comfort measures for pain.

        (5) Promote maternal-infant attachment.

      d) Nursing evaluation

        (1) Infection is identified and appropriately treated.

        (2) Client is comfortable and able to bond with infant.

   C. Infection of the urinary tract (UTI)

     1. Definition: contamination of the urinary tract caused by overdistention, incomplete emptying of the bladder, and catheterization

     2. Risk factors: cervicitis, vaginitis, obstruction of the flaccid ureters, vesicoureteral reflux, bladder trauma resulting from childbirth, catheterization, general anesthesia, cesarean delivery, use of forceps or vacuum extractor

     3. Medical therapy: drainage of overdistended bladder with catheter and administration of antibiotics

     4. Essential nursing care

      a) Nursing assessment

        (1) Monitor for bladder distention.

        (2) Observe for symptoms of infection such as urinary frequency and urgency, dysuria, nocturia, hematuria, suprapubic pain, temperature elevation, and abdominal pain.

      b) Nursing diagnoses

        (1) High risk for infection related to urinary stasis

        (2) Pain related to dysuria secondary to cystitis

        (3) Knowledge deficit related to self-care measures to prevent UTI

      c) Nursing intervention

        (1) Encourage client to void regularly.

        (2) Provide comfort measures (analgesia and ice packs).

        (3) Use aseptic technique for catheterization.

        (4) Instruct client in self-care measures to prevent UTI (see Client Teaching Checklist, "Self-Care Measures to Prevent Urinary Tract Infection").

        d) Nursing evaluation
           (1) Signs of infection are detected early, and condition is treated effectively.
           (2) Client practices appropriate self-care measures to prevent the recurrence of infection.

D. Mastitis
    1. Definition: infection of breast of a breastfeeding mother; usually caused by *Staphylococcus aureus*
    2. Risk factors: poor milk drainage, lowered maternal defenses, poor hygiene, nipple tissue damage
    3. Medical therapy: bed rest; increased fluid intake; abscess drainage; supportive bra; frequent infant feeding; administration of heat, analgesia, and antibiotics
    4. Essential nursing care
        a) Nursing assessment
           (1) Assess client for predisposing factors such as cracked nipples, poor hygiene, and engorgement.
           (2) Observe breasts for consistency, color, surface temperature, and nipple condition.
        b) Nursing diagnoses
           (1) Knowledge deficit related to appropriate breastfeeding techniques
           (2) Pain related to tissue trauma
           (3) Altered parenting related to pain
        c) Nursing intervention
           (1) Teach proper breastfeeding techniques such as complete breast emptying and prevention of cracked nipples.
           (2) Teach client signs and symptoms of mastitis, which usually occur after hospital discharge (e.g., fever; chills; malaise; tenderness, swelling, redness, and warmth in breast).
           (3) Identify cause of mastitis promptly.

    (4) Administer antibiotics as ordered and assist in draining abscesses.

    (5) Help client maintain lactation and relieve engorged breasts if breastfeeding is continued.

   d) Nursing evaluation

    (1) Client is aware of preventive measures.

    (2) Mastitis is detected early and treated promptly.

  E. Thromboembolism

   1. Definition: disorder caused by blood clot that lodges in a blood vessel and obstructs the flow of blood

   2. Types

    a) Thrombophlebitis: thrombus forms on a vessel wall in response to inflammation

    b) Pulmonary embolism: thrombus breaks away from vessel wall (embolus) and is carried by venous circulation to the pulmonary artery

   3. Risk factors: obesity, increased maternal age, high parity, previous history of thrombosis, prolonged inactivity due to anesthesia and surgery, varicosities

   4. Medical therapy: administration of heparin (anticoagulant), antibiotic, and local heat; limb elevation; bed rest; analgesia

   5. Essential nursing care

    a) Nursing assessment

     (1) Identify at-risk clients by assessing for predisposing factors.

     (2) Assess client for positive Homan's sign (pain in leg or foot when leg is extended and foot is dorsiflexed) and for pain in inguinal area or lower abdomen.

    b) Nursing diagnoses

     (1) High risk for injury related to obstructed venous return

     (2) Pain related to tissue hypoxia and edema

     (3) Knowledge deficit related to condition, its treatment, and preventive measures

     (4) Altered parenting related to decreased maternal-infant interaction

    c) Nursing intervention

     (1) Monitor vital signs.

     (2) Maintain bed rest and leg elevation.

     (3) Provide warm, moist soaks.

     (4) Administer IV heparin as ordered, monitor coagulation studies, and observe for signs of overdose.

     (5) Observe for and report promptly signs of pulmonary embolism (see Nurse Alert, "Signs of Pulmonary Embolism").

- Sudden onset of severe chest pain
- Shortness of breath
- Anxiety
- Cough
- Hemoptysis
- Signs of shock: tachycardia, hypotension, diaphoresis, pallor
- Syncope

      (6) Administer analgesia as ordered.

      (7) Promote mother-infant attachment.

   d) Nursing evaluation

      (1) Client recovers fully, and further injury is avoided.

      (2) Secondary bleeding from anticoagulation therapy is avoided.

      (3) Analgesics relieve pain.

      (4) Client bonds successfully with infant.

II. Psychologic problems

┌─────────────────┐
│ See text pages │
│ ───────────── │
└─────────────────┘

A. Postpartum depression

  1. Definition: emotional problems that occur during the postpartum period

  2. Types

    a) "Baby blues"

    b) Neurotic depression

    c) Borderline depression

    d) Psychotic depression

  3. Risk factors: previous puerperal depression, maternal history of manic-depressive illness, substance abuse, lack of stable relationship, lack of social support, low socioeconomic status, obsessive personality

  4. Treatment: support, information, reassurance, psychotherapy, medication, hospitalization

  5. Essential nursing care

    a) Nursing assessment

      (1) Identify at-risk clients.

      (2) Observe for signs and symptoms of depression in the postpartum period.

    b) Nursing diagnoses

      (1) Ineffective individual coping related to postpartum depression

      (2) Altered parenting related to impaired bonding

       c) Nursing intervention

         (1) Educate client and family about the possibility of postpartum depression, and reassure them of its short-term nature.

         (2) Provide support, and encourage client to express her feelings.

         (3) Encourage client to see mental health professional for counseling.

         (4) Assist client and family in obtaining household help and infant care.

         (5) Arrange for possible postpartum follow-up after discharge.

       d) Nursing evaluation

         (1) Signs of postpartum depression are detected early, and therapy is initiated.

         (2) Alternative care is provided until client is able to care for infant.

B. Failure to bond

  1. Definition: poorly developed attachment between caregiver and infant resulting in inadequate responses to the infant

  2. Risk factors

    a) Abnormal pregnancy, labor, or birth

    b) Substance abuse

    c) Separation of infant and caregiver within first 6 months

    d) Neonatal or maternal illness in first 12 months

    e) Any situation that postpones maternal or paternal contact

  3. Treatment: use of team approach, incorporating all nursing shifts as well as community resources

  4. Essential nursing care

    a) Nursing assessment

      (1) Identify at-risk client in prenatal period.

      (2) Identify promptly any maladaptive parental behaviors (see Nurse Alert, "Warning Signs of Impaired Bonding").

    b) Nursing diagnoses

      (1) Altered family processes related to addition of new infant

      (2) Knowledge deficit related to emotional needs of newborn

      (3) Altered parenting related to separation of high-risk newborn and parents

    c) Nursing intervention

      (1) Provide information about needs of newborn.

      (2) Encourage positive behaviors demonstrated by parents.

      (3) Investigate modifying hospital routine to allow increased contact with infant.

        (4) Provide support and understanding.

        (5) Make appropriate community referrals and provide postdischarge follow-up.

    d) Nursing evaluation

        (1) Client demonstrates appropriate interaction with infant.

        (2) Client makes use of community resources for ongoing support and counseling.

C. Loss of fetus or newborn and threat of loss of high-risk infant: essential nursing care

  1. Nursing assessment

    a) Determine nature of loss or potential loss and client's response.

    b) Explore individual circumstances of client and family.

        (1) Past grief experiences

        (2) Religious and cultural beliefs

        (3) Age and maturity level of parents

        (4) Family support system

        (5) Usual coping methods in crisis

  2. Nursing diagnoses

    a) Knowledge deficit related to perinatal loss

    b) Knowledge deficit related to the grieving process

    c) Ineffective individual (or family) coping related to death of fetus/neonate or client

    d) Altered family processes/parenting related to loss

    e) Spiritual distress related to loss

! NURSE _ALERT_ !

Warning Signs of Impaired Bonding

Maternal behaviors
- Lack of interest in infant
- Negative comments about infant's appearance
- Limited or no eye contact with infant
- Limited handling of infant
- Holding infant away from body
- Handling infant without stroking face or extremities
- Lack of preparation for infant care at home

Paternal behaviors
- Rough, unrelaxed handling of infant
- Lack of interest in infant
- Inappropriate play
- Lack of protective attitude toward infant

    3. Nursing intervention

       a) Provide information on the circumstances of the loss and prepare family for time with the infant.

       b) Encourage family to discuss feelings.

       c) Encourage parents to visit high-risk infant as much as possible.

       d) Anticipate and provide information on the different stages of the grieving process.

       e) Provide support and reassurance to client and family throughout the grieving process.

       f) Assist with the parents' decision making (notify clergy, prepare funeral, name infant).

       g) Make referrals to appropriate community support groups.

    4. Nursing evaluation

       a) Parents understand the grieving process and are able to be supportive of one another.

       b) Parents are able to verbalize their feelings.

       c) Parents understand prognosis for high-risk infant.

       d) Parents feel supported by hospital staff and make use of appropriate community resources.

1. The first sign of early postpartum hemorrhage is:

   a. Uterine atony.
   b. Hypotension.
   c. Weakness.
   d. Oliguria.

2. Merilie, who is postpartum day 1, is receiving early discharge teaching from the nurse. What statement by Merilie indicates a correct understanding of danger signs that she should report to her health care provider?

   a. "If I saturate more than one peripad an hour, I should call my caregiver."
   b. "If my temperature is 100°F, I should call my caregiver."
   c. "If my vaginal discharge turns brown, I should contact my caregiver."
   d. "I should contact my caregiver when my menstrual period begins."

3. Mrs. Wagner, who is postpartum day 2, tells the nurse that she has increasing abdomen tenderness and chills. Her temperature is 102.4°F. Upon examination, the nurse assesses foul-smelling lochia. Mrs. Wagner most likely has:

   a. Retained placenta.
   b. Endometritis.
   c. Mastitis.
   d. Episiotomy abscess.

4. The most common cause of puerperal reproductive tract infection is:

   a. *Neisseria gonorrhoeae.*
   b. *Pseudomonas aeruginosa.*
   c. *Candida albicans.*
   d. Group B beta-hemolytic streptococcus.

5. While assessing a postpartum client, the nurse notes pain, warmth, and swelling in the right calf and a positive Homan's sign. The nurse interprets this to be:

   a. Pain related to tissue hypoxia and edema.

   b. High risk for injury related to hemorrhage.
   c. High risk for injury related to infection.
   d. Decreased cardiac output related to reduced coagulation.

6. A client receiving heparin therapy for thromboembolitic disease should be closely monitored for:

   a. Dehydration.
   b. Epistaxis.
   c. Hemolytic anemia.
   d. Hyperprothrombinemia.

7. Should a client demonstrate signs of heparin overdose, the nurse should expect the physician to order:

   a. Warfarin sodium.
   b. Promethazine hydrochloride.
   c. Pentazocine lactate.
   d. Protamine sulfate.

8. To prevent overdistention of the bladder, the nurse should encourage the postpartum woman to:

   a. Restrict fluid intake.
   b. Void frequently.
   c. Self-catheterize every 4 hours.
   d. Massage bladder prior to voiding.

9. A common contributing factor for mastitis in the breastfeeding mother is:

   a. Inadequate fluid intake.
   b. Cracked nipples.
   c. Inverted nipples.
   d. Breast shields.

10. Lola delivered an 8-lb baby girl at 8:10 A.M. As of 6 P.M., she has not voided. Lola states that she has no urge to void. Physical assessment reveals a full bladder. The best nursing action to take is to:

    a. Increase the client's fluid intake.
    b. Pour warm water over the perineum.
    c. Catheterize the client.
    d. Provide a diuretic.

11. Which of the following statements would alert the nurse to the potential for impaired bonding between mother and child?

    a. "You have your daddy's eyes."
    b. "Your bowel movements are so disgusting."
    c. "Where did he get all that hair?"
    d. "He seems to sleep too much."

12. Baby Girl J was born at 28 weeks' gestation and died of complications related to respiratory distress syndrome. To assist the parents in validating their loss, the nurse should:

    a. Assist the parents in making funeral arrangements.
    b. Refer the parents to a support group.
    c. Inform the staff members to leave the parents alone.
    d. Encourage the parents to hold their dead baby.

ANSWERS

1. Correct answer is a. Uterine atony, or relaxation of the uterus, is the initial sign of postpartum hemorrhage. This is assessed as a boggy or soft uterus.

    b. Signs of hypotension may not be seen until there is a large amount of blood loss. This is due to increased blood volume in the postpartum woman.
    c. Weakness may be present with hemorrhage, but most postpartum women experience weakness. This would not be an initial sign of hemorrhage.
    d. Oliguria would be a later sign of hemorrhage.

2. Correct answer is a. Saturating more than one peripad an hour suggests postpartum hemorrhage, and the client should call her caregiver.

    b. A temperature of 100°F does not warrant a call to the caregiver. Should it rise to 101°F, the caregiver should be notified.
    c. The normal involution process progresses lochia from red to pink to brown.
    d. The caregiver does not need to be notified of the return of menses.

3. Correct answer is b. The symptoms presented would strongly suggest endometritis.

    a. Hemorrhage and uterine atony are signs of retained placenta.
    c. Mastitis is infection of the breasts. The client does not present with symptoms of mastitis except for elevated temperature and chills.
    d. Abdominal pain and discharge would not be consistent with an abscessed episiotomy.

4. Correct answer is d. Group B beta-hemolytic streptococcus is the most common cause of postpartum infection of the woman's reproductive tract.

    a. *Neisseria gonorrhoeae* may cause postpartum infection, but it is not the most common cause.
    b. *Pseudomonas* rarely causes postpartum infection.
    c. *Candida albicans* is a yeastlike fungus that is commonly seen during pregnancy. However, it would be an unlikely cause of a postpartum infection.

5. Correct answer is a. The data presented support pain caused by tissue hypoxia and edema. This strongly suggests a deep vein thrombosis (DVT).

    b. High risk for injury related to hemorrhage is inappropriate since a hemorrhage is not a classic sign of DVT.
    c. The data presented do not imply infection.
    d. There are no data here to support decreased cardiac output.

6. **Correct answer is b.** Signs of heparin overdose result in bleeding, including hematuria, epistaxis, ecchymosis, and bleeding gums.

   a. Dehydration is not normally seen in heparin therapy.
   c. Hemolytic anemia is caused by the increased destruction of erythrocytes. This is not related to heparin therapy.
   d. Anticoagulation therapy has a hypoprothrombinemic effect. Hyperprothombinemia would be an unusual action and highly unlikely.

7. **Correct answer is d.** Protamine sulfate is a heparin antagonist.

   a. Warfarin sodium is also an anticoagulant.
   b. Promethazine hydrochloride is an antihistamine and would not be used for heparin overdose.
   c. Pentazocine lactate is an analgesic and would not be used to treat heparin overdose.

8. **Correct answer is b.** The postpartum woman should be encouraged to void frequently in order to prevent bladder distention.

   a. Fluids should not be restricted in the postpartum period since diaphoresis is common.
   c. There is no need to self-catheterize.
   d. Massaging the bladder will not prevent overdistention.

9. **Correct answer is b.** Cracked nipples provide a portal of entry for microorganisms and thus can contribute to mastitis.

   a and c. Inadequate fluid intake and inverted nipples are not contributing factors for mastitis.
   d. If worn correctly and removed as directed, breast shields do not lead to mastitis.

10. **Correct answer is c.** A client should void by 6 hours postdelivery. Because this client is 10 hours postdelivery and has no urge to urinate, straight catheterization is the appropriate action.

    a. Increasing a client's fluid intake will not stimulate urination.
    b. Pouring warm water over the perineum is sometimes helpful to stimulate urination. However, because this client is 10 hours postdelivery, it is important that she empty her bladder immediately in order to prevent complications.
    d. This is not an appropriate nursing action; a diuretic requires a physician's order. Also, it is not the appropriate therapy.

11. **Correct answer is b.** Negative comments about the infant's appearance, behavior, and excreta are all warning signs of possible impaired bonding.

    a, c, and **d.** Questioning and comparing the infant's characteristics are part of the normal process of bonding and attachment.

12. **Correct answer is d.** Validating loss is promoted by having the parents and family view and hold the dead child.

    a. Assisting the parents in making funeral arrangements provides the family with needed support but does not directly relate to validating their loss.
    b. Referral to a support group may not be appropriate at this time. It would not necessarily validate their loss.
    c. At the time of death, parents need the support of family and staff. Parents may be provided with private space, but staff should stay close by for support if the parents wish.

Maternal-Newborn Comprehensive Review Questions

1. Sarah is a single parent with 2 children. Sarah's mother also lives with her. This is an example of a(n):
   a. Extended family.
   b. Nuclear family.
   c. Kin network.
   d. Single-adult family.

2. Which of the following attributes of cervical mucus helps signify the onset of ovulation?
   a. Mucus becomes thick, cloudy, and viscous.
   b. Mucus is thin, clear, and stretchable.
   c. Mucus amount decreases.
   d. Mucus becomes yellowish in color.

3. Embryonic membranes and germ layers form during the preembryonic stage of human development. The endoderm germ layer eventually forms the:
   a. Epidermis and nervous system.
   b. Bone and cartilage.
   c. Respiratory and digestive tracts.
   d. Blood, blood vessels, and pericardium.

4. In fetal circulation, fetal blood bypasses the fetal lungs. The bypass structure is called the:
   a. Ductus arteriosus.
   b. Ductus venosus.
   c. Inferior vena cava.
   d. Descending aorta.

5. Everett and Mary have been trying to achieve pregnancy for the past year and are now seeking medical advice. Everett has been asked to bring a semen specimen to the Fertility Clinic for analysis. The nurse should give him the following information:
   a. Specimen should be collected after having sexual intercourse for 4 consecutive days.
   b. If specimen is collected during intercourse, a condom lubricated with nonoxynol 9 should be used.
   c. Specimen should be stored in a refrigerator until brought to the clinic.
   d. Specimen should be brought to the clinic in a clean, dry glass or plastic container within 1–3 hours of collection.

6. Ms. Choy, at 10 weeks' gestation, is scheduled for an abortion. What type of abortion procedure would most probably be done at this point in Ms. Choy's first trimester?
   a. Hypertonic saline
   b. Vacuum curettage
   c. Menstrual extraction
   d. Prostaglandin E_2 suppositories

7. The nurse is leading a childbirth preparation class. One of the members of the group is Deb, age 15. The best teaching method for the nurse to use to facilitate Deb's understanding of the breathing techniques during labor is:
   a. Reading material.
   b. A videotape.
   c. Practice sessions.
   d. Group discussion.

8. The nurse is evaluating a client's knowledge of warning signs during pregnancy. Which statement by the client indicates a correct understanding of warning signs?
   a. "If I have urinary frequency, I should contact the physician."
   b. "I need to report any fatigue I am experiencing."
   c. "I should call the clinic if I have blurred or double vision."
   d. "Any shortness of breath should be reported immediately."

9. Le Wong, age 18 and at 22 weeks' gestation, complains to the nurse that she has increasing fatigue and swelling in her ankles by noon. Upon examination, the nurse finds Le's urine protein 2+, weight gain of 4 lb since her visit 1 month ago, and blood pressure of 138/92. The nurse interprets these signs as:

   a. HELLP syndrome.
   b. Hypertensive crisis.
   c. Eclampsia.
   d. Preeclampsia.

10. While assessing a client with preeclampsia who is receiving magnesium sulfate ($MgSO_4$) intravenously, the nurse observes an absence of patellar reflex and a respiratory rate of 12/minute. The first nursing action should be to:

   a. Call the physician.
   b. Give calcium gluconate.
   c. Stop the $MgSO_4$ infusion.
   d. Start oxygen per nasal cannula.

11. While monitoring fetal heart tones in a client who is in active labor, the nurse notes early decelerations. The nurse should:

   a. Start oxygen at 10 l/minute by mask.
   b. Continue to monitor fetal heart tones.
   c. Change maternal position.
   d. Notify the physician immediately.

12. Using Leopold's maneuvers on a client in the labor room, the nurse assesses the fetal position to be left occipitoanterior (LOA). In this position, the fetal heart tones can be best heard in which quadrant of the maternal abdomen?

   a. Right upper quadrant
   b. Left upper quadrant
   c. Right lower quadrant
   d. Left lower quadrant

13. While electronically monitoring fetal heart tones during a client's first stage of labor, the nurse notes moderate to severe variable decelerations and suspects cord prolapse. The nurse should place the client in which of the following positions?

   a. Knee-chest position
   b. Dorsal-recumbent position
   c. Semi-Fowler's position
   d. Upright position

14. For which of the following laboring or postpartum clients would oxytocin be contraindicated?

   a. Helen: postpartum bleeding
   b. Lois: prolonged labor
   c. Portia: active genital herpes infection
   d. Tawanda: type I diabetes

15. Newborn Baby Girl A is being monitored for respiratory distress related to an IV narcotic analgesic given to the mother for labor pains 30 minutes before delivery. The nurse caring for Baby Girl A should have readily available:

   a. A radiant warmer.
   b. Intravenous dextrose.
   c. Naloxone (Narcan).
   d. DeLee mucus trap.

16. The nurse needs to obtain a blood sample from Newborn Baby Girl F for a glucose level. The best place for a needlestick in a newborn is the:

   a. Femoral artery.
   b. Medial aspect of the heel.
   c. Lateral aspect of the heel.
   d. Plantar surface of the foot.

17. Baby Girl D was born 1 hour ago. Her mother has type I diabetes. The nurse is aware that the newborn is at high risk for hypoglycemia. Initial signs of neonatal hypoglycemia include:

   a. Lethargy.
   b. Jaundice.
   c. Seizure.
   d. Acrocyanosis.

18. To prevent hypoglycemia in Baby Girl D, the nurse should:
    a. Give only water.
    b. Administer a 25%–50% dextrose infusion.
    c. Administer corticosteroids.
    d. Encourage early breast or formula feeding.

19. Baby Boy T is born with fetal alcohol syndrome (FAS). To facilitate effective feeding and promote weight gain, the nurse should:
    a. Gavage feed the infant.
    b. Allow extra time during feeding.
    c. Initiate total parenteral nutrition (TPN).
    d. Prop the bottle on a pillow.

20. Which of the following women is most at risk for bearing a baby with intrauterine growth retardation (IUGR)?
    a. Liz, age 25, gravida 3 para 2
    b. Julia, age 31, rheumatoid arthritis
    c. Clara, age 16, smoker
    d. Abby, age 21, hepatitis B carrier

21. Sherry, who is 2 days postpartum, has bright-red vaginal discharge with many small clots. This is called:
    a. Lochia alba.
    b. Lochia serosa.
    c. Lochia rubra.
    d. Lochia purulenta.

22. The postpartum nurse reviewing the labor and delivery record of Amy discovers that Amy had a prolonged second stage of labor and extended periods of time in the stirrups. The postpartum nurse interprets this to mean that Amy is at high risk for:
    a. Retained placenta.
    b. Hypertension.
    c. Diastasis recti abdominis.
    d. Thrombophlebitis.

23. Molly, age 16, had a pregnancy weight gain of 15 lb and iron deficiency anemia. She failed to show for more than half of her scheduled prenatal visits. Her labor was prolonged, and she delivered a 6-lb infant by cesarean section. During the postpartum period, Molly is at risk for:
    a. Hemorrhage.
    b. Postpartum depression.
    c. Infections.
    d. Dehydration.

24. While completing newborn care teaching with a new mother who is postpartum day 2, the nurse observes that the mother is anxious and irritable and has difficulty concentrating. The mother begins to cry and states, "I'll never remember all of this. I don't think I'll make a very good mother." Based on these data, the nurse interprets this behavior as most likely:
    a. Altered parenting related to impaired bonding.
    b. Knowledge deficit related to emotional and physical needs of newborn.
    c. Situational low self-esteem related to knowledge deficits and postpartum blues.
    d. Altered family processes related to addition of a new infant.

ANSWERS

1. **Correct answer is a.** An extended family is one in which one or more grandparents live with a single-parent family or a nuclear family.
    b. Nuclear family refers to husband, wife, and children who live in a common household.
    c. Kin network refers to 2 or more nuclear families or unmarried households living in close proximity.
    d. Single-adult family refers to an unmarried adult living alone.

2. Correct answer is b. This type of mucus is a result of estrogen effects. Mucus that is thin, clear, and elastic promotes sperm viability.

a. Cervical mucus becomes thick, cloudy, and viscous under the influence of progesterone after ovulation.
c. Mucus amount increases right before ovulation.
d. Cervical mucus should be clear to white in color regardless of the phase of ovarian cycle. A change to yellow may indicate a medical problem.

3. Correct answer is c. The endoderm, or inner germ layer, forms the respiratory and digestive tracts as well as the bladder and urethra.

a. The ectoderm, or outer layer, forms the epidermis, nervous system, external sense organs, and mucous membranes of mouth and anus.
b and d. The mesoderm, or middle layer, forms the connective tissue, bone, cartilage, muscle, blood and blood vessels, kidneys, lymphatics, gonads, pericardium, and peritoneum.

4. Correct answer is a. Both the ductus arteriosus and the foramen ovale act as bypass channels, allowing cardiac output to return to the placenta without flowing through the lungs.

b. The ductus venosus carries blood to the inferior vena cava.
c. The inferior vena cava brings venous blood to the right atrium, which then flows through the foramen ovale.
d. The aorta receives blood from the ductus arteriosus.

5. Correct answer is d. Clients should be taught to place semen specimen in a clean, dry glass or plastic container. To ensure the best specimen possible, client should bring it to the clinic within 1–3 hours after collection.

a. Specimen should be collected after abstaining from sex for 2–3 days.
b. Condoms may be used for collection of specimen. However, no spermicidal agents should be used.
c. Specimen must be kept at body temperature during transport to clinic. This can be done by carrying it under the arm.

6. Correct answer is b. A vacuum curettage is the most common type of abortion procedure in the first trimester. It is often accompanied by insertion of laminaria prior to the procedure to facilitate cervical dilatation.

a and d. Both are used in second-trimester abortions.
c. Menstrual extractions are done very early in pregnancy, usually within 2 weeks of missed period.

7. Correct answer is c. Adolescents are concrete learners and do best with specific examples and practice sessions to reinforce learning.

a. Adolescents do not assimilate written material as well as direct practice.
b. A videotape would be well received by an adolescent, but practice would still be needed to reinforce learning.
d. Group discussions may be difficult for an adolescent, especially if there are no peers in the group.

8. Correct answer is c. Blurred or double vision or spots before the eyes are a danger sign and may indicate hypertension or preeclampsia.

a. Urinary frequency is common during pregnancy due to the increased uterine size placing pressure on the bladder.
b. Fatigue is a normal aspect of pregnancy.
d. Shortness of breath is common as the pregnancy advances. This is due to the increased uterine size exerting pressure on the diaphragm.

9. **Correct answer is d.** The three cardinal signs of preeclampsia are hypertension, edema, and proteinuria.

a. HELLP syndrome is multiple organ failure (i.e., hemolysis, elevated liver enzymes, and low platelet count).
b. Hypertensive crisis in pregnancy exists when maternal blood pressure is 160/110. It is associated with PIH and chronic hypertension.
c. Eclampsia refers to a progression from preeclampsia when the clinical course includes convulsions.

10. **Correct answer is c.** The manifestations presented are those of $MgSO_4$ toxicity. The first action should be to stop the cause of the toxicity.

a. The physician should be notified after initial emergency measures are instituted.
b. Calcium gluconate is the appropriate antagonist to give once the $MgSO_4$ has been stopped.
d. Oxygen may or may not be given, depending on other variables.

11. **Correct answer is b.** Early decelerations are considered normal and benign. They are a response to compression of the fetal head by uterine contractions and do not indicate fetal distress. The nurse would need to continue to monitor fetal heart tones as per routine.

a and d. These actions are inappropriate because this is not an emergency situation in which fetal distress is indicated. Oxygen is not needed nor would the physician need to be notified at this time.
c. A change in maternal position would not affect early decelerations.

12. **Correct answer is d.** In the left occipitoanterior, the fetal heart tones are heard best in maternal left lower quadrant.

a. Fetal heart tones heard in right upper quadrant may indicate RSA (right sacroanterior) position.
b. Fetal heart tones heard in left upper quadrant may indicate LSA (left sacroanterior) position.

c. Fetal heart tones heard in right lower quadrant include ROP (right occipitoposterior) and ROA (right occipitoanterior) positions.

13. **Correct answer is a.** The knee-chest position allows gravity to relieve compression on the cord.

b. The dorsal-recumbent, or supine, position would be contraindicated because it causes a decrease in placental perfusion.
c and d. Neither the semi-Fowler's position nor the upright position would be beneficial when the cord has prolapsed.

14. **Correct answer is c.** A client with active genital herpes is not a candidate for a vaginal delivery. Thus, oxytocin would be contraindicated.

a, b, and **d.** Oxytocin is not contraindicated for postpartum bleeding, prolonged labor, or type I diabetes.

15. **Correct answer is c.** Should Baby Girl A experience respiratory distress as a result of maternal narcotic analgesia, the appropriate nursing action would be to administer naloxone (Narcan), which is a narcotic antagonist.

a. A radiant warmer may be necessary to stabilize temperature, but the first priority is the newborn's respiratory stability.
b. IV dextrose would not normally be required.
d. A DeLee mucus trap is one method of suctioning a newborn. However, Baby Girl A's primary difficulty is the effects of narcotic analgesic, which can be reversed with naloxone.

16. **Correct answer is c.** The lateral aspect of the heel is free of arteries and nerves.

a. The femoral artery is an inappropriate site for obtaining blood for a blood glucose test.
b. The medial aspect of the heel is not appropriate because of the location of the medial calcaneal nerves and medial plantar artery.
d. The plantar surface is not appropriate because the medial and lateral plantar nerves are located there.

17. **Correct answer is a.** Lethargy may be seen in the neonate with hypoglycemia. This relates to lack of glucose to nerve cells with subsequent CNS changes.

   b. Jaundice is not a sign of hypoglycemia.
   c. Seizure is not an initial sign of hypoglycemia. It is a late CNS symptom.
   d. Acrocyanosis is a normal physiologic process in the newborn related to immature capillary function.

18. **Correct answer is d.** This infant would greatly benefit from early feeding so that glucose levels remain above hypoglycemia level.

   a. Giving only water could lead to even lower glucose levels.
   b. An infusion of 25%–50% dextrose is contraindicated because it may cause rebound hypoglycemia; 5%–10% glucose is used.
   c. Corticosteroids are not a prevention measure. They are used, however, in severe cases of hypoglycemia to promote gluconeogenesis from noncarbohydrate proteins.

19. **Correct answer is b.** The newborn with FAS is difficult to feed. He may have poor sucking, disinterest in feeding, and persistent vomiting. The nurse feeding this newborn needs to be patient and allow extra time for feedings.

   a. The infant should not be gavage fed unless he fails to take adequate formula from a bottle.
   c. TPN would not be appropriate unless the infant has significant inability to digest nutrients. This is not normally the case with FAS.
   d. It is always inappropriate to prop an infant's bottle on a pillow.

20. **Correct answer is c.** Both her young age and the fact that she smokes put Clara at a high risk for IUGR.

   a. Liz's parity status does not indicate high risk for IUGR.

   b. Rheumatoid arthritis in and of itself does not predispose for IUGR. However, if the woman takes large amounts of salicylates, their teratogenic effect may lead to IUGR.
   d. Pregnant women who are hepatitis B carriers have no greater risk for IUGR than the general population.

21. **Correct answer is c.** Postpartum lochia that is bright red with small clots is called lochia rubra. This occurs for 1–3 days postpartum.

   a. Lochia alba occurs 1–3 weeks postpartum and is light cream to brownish in color.
   b. Lochia serosa is pink to pinkish brown and contains degenerating blood cells and endometrium. It contains no clots. It occurs 4–7 days postpartum.
   d. Lochia purulenta is another name for lochia alba.

22. **Correct answer is d.** Prolonged pressure on the lower extremities that occurred because Amy was positioned in stirrups for a prolonged period, as well as clotting changes that occur during the postpartum period, puts Amy at a high risk for thrombophlebitis.

   a. A retained placenta may or may not relate to the length of the second stage of labor.
   b. Hypertension does not necessarily relate to a prolonged second stage of labor.
   c. Relaxation or separation of the abdominal muscles does not relate to a prolonged second stage of labor.

23. **Correct answer is c.** A poor nutritional status and lack of prenatal care combined with a prolonged labor and subsequent cesarean section identify this client as being at risk for infections.

   a. Client is no more at risk for hemorrhage than any other postpartum client.
   b. Given the data provided, this client has the same risk for postpartum depression as any other client.
   d. This client has no more of a risk for dehydration than any other postpartum client.

24. **Correct answer is c.** The client is showing symptoms of low self-esteem that are related to postpartum blues and inability to remember or understand the teaching. This is situational in nature.

a. There are no data presented to support impaired bonding.

b. The data presented do not totally support a knowledge deficit.

d. There is only one statement by the client that may indicate a *potential* altered family process but not the actual problem.